Alkaline Diet Cookbook

400 Recipes For Rapid Weight Loss & Balancing Your pH Levels

Gloria Lee

© Copyright 2017 by Gloria Lee - All Rights Reserved.

Under no circumstances can any piece of information in this book be republished or quoted without direct permission from the author.

Disclaimer:

This book is intended for entertainment and information purposes only. The author and any other creators of this book are in no way liable or hold any responsibility for the adverse effects that you may take from directly or indirectly reading this book. It's advised that you seek a medical professional if you plan on altering your diet or taking up any health related practice.

Table of Contents

Introduction 11

BREAKFAST RECIPES 12

1 - Breakfast Quinoa Salad 12
2 - Carrot & Pineapple Cake Oatmeal 12
3 - Warming Stew 13
4 - Sweet Potato Avocado Toasts 13
5 - Smoky Sweet Potato & Kale Hash 13
6 - Chopped Breakfast Salad 14
7 - Chai Spiced Breakfast Quinoa 14
8 - Chia Energy Parfait 14
9 - Warm Apple Pie Breakfast Cereal 15
10 - Southwest Tofu Scramble 15
11 - Fruity Chia Pots 15
12 - Sweet Potato Parfait 16
13 - Broccoli & Tofu Sandwich 16
14 - Nutty Overnight Oats 16
15 - Sunnyside Breakfast Bowl 17
16 - Turmeric Oats 17
17 - Alkaline Breakfast Raw Mix 17
18 - Mexican Breakfast Bowl 18
19 - Avocado Zucchini Toast 18
20 - Savory Asian Oatmeal 19
21 - Breakfast Fruit Crepes 19
22 - Cabbage & Potato Hash 19
23 - Mediterranean Tofu Scramble 20
24 - Tomato Toast 20
25 - Spicy Tofu Breakfast Bake 20
26 - Coconut Granola 21
27 - Beet Breakfast Hash 21
28 - Citrus Breakfast Salad 21
29 - Turmeric Citrus Crepes 22
30 - Sweet Almond Pears 22
31 - Berry Oatmeal 22
32 - Tropical Chia Bowl 23
33 - Sunshine Granola & Kefir 23
34 - Sweet Potato & Zucchini Hash Brown 24
35 - Nutty Breakfast Squash 24
36 - Spicy Avocado Breakfast Boat 25
37 - Brussel Sprout Hash 25
38 - Garden Chickpea Omelet 26
39 - Mocha Pudding 26
40 - Chocolate Chia Breakfast 27
41 - Zippy Ginger Breakfast Bars 27
42 - Breakfast Squash Bread 27
43 - Cherry Almond Bake 28
44 - Salmon & Cabbage Hash 28
45 - Summer Medley Parfait 28
46 - Mexican Breakfast Toast 29
47 - Omega- Overnight Oats 29
48 - Broccoli Omelet 29
49 - Tofu & Kale Tacos 30
50 - Fruit Porridge 30
51 - Morning Sweet Bread 30
52 - Banana Breakfast Pudding 31
53 - Italian Breakfast Hash 31
54 - Papaya Breakfast Boat 31

55 - AM Quinoa Cookies ... 32
56 - Savory Breakfast Bowl ... 32
57 - Almond Butter & Jelly Overnight Oats ... 33
58 - Broccoli & Sprouts Savory Oats ... 33
59 - Fruit & Millet Breakfast ... 33
60 - Avocado Breakfast Soup ... 34
61 - Sweet Orange Oats ... 34

APPETIZER/SNACKS RECIPES ... 35

62 - Greek Zucchini Cups ... 35
63 - Endive & Watercress Boats ... 35
64 - Toasted Trail Mix ... 35
65 - Chickpea Avocado Cups ... 35
66 - Spicy Cocoa-Coco Truffles ... 36
67 - Adult Ants on a Log ... 36
68 - Asian Cucumber Slaw ... 36
69 - Broiled Grapefruit ... 36
70 - Coconut Curry Soup ... 37
71 - Chilled Avocado Cilantro Soup ... 37
72 - Cooling Cucumber Slice Snack ... 38
73 - Spicy Tortilla Soup ... 38
74 - Raw Green Gazpacho ... 38
75 - Zesty Green Chips ... 39
76 - Mediterranean Spread ... 39
77 - Summer Fruit Soup ... 39
78 - Carrot Tahini Slaw ... 40
79 - Veggie Chips ... 40
80 - Spiced Middle Eastern Dip ... 40
81 - Detox Soup ... 41
82 - Vegetarian Paté ... 41
83 - Sage & Butternut Squash Soup ... 41
84 - Chilled Tomato Soup ... 42
85 - Sweet & Sour Cabbage ... 42
86 - Vegetable & Lentil Soup ... 42
87 - Roasted Red Pepper Dip ... 42
88 - Ghee & Maple Roasted Carrots ... 43
89 - Edamame Salad ... 43
90 - Smokey Caesar Salad ... 43
91 - Baked Sweet Potato Fries with Spicy BBQ Sauce ... 44
92 - Citrus & Jicama Salad ... 44
93 - Green Cabbage Slaw ... 44
94 - Spicy Mix with Tortilla Chips ... 45
95 - Creamy Broccoli Soup ... 45
96 - Chilled Coconut Soup ... 46
97 - Root Vegetable Soup ... 46
98 - Squash Dip with Cucumber Slices ... 46
99 - Creamy Two Bean Salad ... 47
100 - Chilled Beet Soup ... 47
101 - Green Hummus ... 47
102 - Spinach Artichoke Dip ... 48
103 - Spinach Cabbage Soup ... 48
104 - Fermented Greens ... 48
105 - Coconut Asparagus Soup ... 49
106 - Vegetable & Rice Stew ... 49
107 - Dairy Free Fruity Milk Jar ... 49
108 - Cleansing Soup ... 49
109 - Red Citrus Salad ... 50
110 - Sweet Summer Soup ... 50
111 - Melon Pie ... 50
112 - Super Smooth Parsnip Soup ... 51

113 - Cucumber & Salmon Cups	51
114 - Sweet Sweet Potato Toasts	52
115 - Eggplant Cashew Bites	52
116 - Curry Chips	52
117 - Mexican Dip	53
118 - Three Onion Soup	53
119 - Watermelon, Mint & Tofu Kebabs	53
120 - Blackberry Salsa	54
121 - Smokey Nut Mix	54
122 - Seaweed Spread	54
123 - Spring Soup	55
124 - Herbed Mushrooms	55
125 - Guacamole Hummus	55
126 - Avocado & Tomato Salad	56
127 - Cheesy Zucchini Chips	56
128 - Curry Pepper Hummus	56
129 - Mushroom & Onion Kebabs	57
130 - Open Faced Avocado Sandwich	57
131 - Mediterranean Parsnip Fries	57
132 - Spicy Sweet Potato Bites	58
133 - Scallion Chickpea Cakes	58
134 - Sweet Chili Carrot Fries	58
135 - Spiced Apple Slices	59
136 - Coconut Butter Dates	59
137 - Warm Avocado Cups	59
138 - Fruit Salsa	59
139 - Chocolate Orange Pineapple Rings	60
140 - Raspberry Mint Yogurt Pops	60
141 - Cheesy Bean Chips	60
142 - Banana Strawberry Bites	61
143 - Spinach & Artichoke Stuffed Mushroom	61
144 - Quick Avocado Wraps	61
145 - Strawberry Toast	62
146 - Triple Berry Parfait	62
147 - Sweet & Savory Almonds	62
148 - Plantain Chips	63
149 - Coconut Figgy Toast	63
150 - Tamari Pepitas Snack	63
151 - Sweet Roasted Chickpeas	63
152 - Roasted Broccoli with Tahini Dip	64

DRINK RECIPES 65

153 - Green Goddess Smoothie	65
154 - Spicy & Smooth Green Shake	65
155 - Tropical Smoothie	65
156 - Ginger Blast Smoothie	65
157 - Spicy Golden Tea	66
158 - Lemon Basil Zinger	66
159 - Bloody Mary Shake	66
160 - Alkaline Veggie Juice	66
161 - Coconut Lime Smoothie	67
162 - Berry Blast Smoothie	67
163 - Minty Morning Shake	67
164 - Green Tea & Fruit Smoothie	67
165 - Apple Pie Smoothie	68
166 - Morning Alkaline Lemon Water	68
167 - Detox Juice	68
168 - Fruity Summer Lemonade	68
169 - All Day Detox Water	69
170 - Watermelon Mint Water	69

- 171 - Glow Juice ... 69
- 172 - Creamy Green Smoothie ... 69
- 173 - Creamy Orange Smoothie ... 70
- 174 - Sunrise Juice ... 70
- 175 - Mulled Cider ... 70
- 176 - Melon Melody ... 70
- 177 - Mango Colada ... 71
- 178 - Herbal Tonic ... 71
- 179 - Probiotic Citrus Drink ... 71
- 180 - Acid Buster Juice ... 71
- 181 - Detox Stimulator Juice ... 72
- 182 - Carrot Dream Smoothie ... 72

LUNCH RECIPES ... 73

- 183 - Southwest Stuffed Sweet Potatoes ... 73
- 184 - Coconut Cauliflower with Herbs & Spices ... 73
- 185 - Zoodles with Avocado Cream Sauce ... 73
- 186 - Rainbow Pad Thai ... 74
- 187 - Creamy Broccoli Slaw ... 74
- 188 - Greek Vegetable Salad ... 74
- 189 - Sweet & Spicy Vegetable Wrap ... 75
- 190 - Mediterranean Millet Salad ... 75
- 191 - Grab & Go Zucchini Rolls ... 76
- 192 - Apple Kale Salad ... 76
- 193 - Lentils & Greens Rice Pilaf ... 77
- 194 - Collard Wraps ... 77
- 195 - Sesame Greens & Tofu ... 77
- 196 - Roasted Carrot & Quinoa Salad ... 78
- 197 - Raw Fennel Salad with Citrus Dressing ... 78
- 198 - Taco Salad Bowl ... 78
- 199 - Veggie & Mango Sushi ... 79
- 200 - Buddha Bowl ... 79
- 201 - Confetti Cauliflower Rice ... 80
- 202 - Creamy Sweet Salad ... 80
- 203 - Sweet Spinach Salad ... 81
- 204 - Creamy Fruit Salad ... 81
- 205 - Steamed Green Bowl ... 81
- 206 - Indian Cauliflower & Potato ... 82
- 207 - Berry & Vegetable Salad ... 82
- 208 - Shredded Cauliflower Salad ... 82
- 209 - Root Vegetable & Citrus Bowl ... 83
- 210 - Veggie Jambalaya ... 83
- 211 - Detox Salad ... 84
- 212 - Alkaline Falafel Salad ... 84
- 213 - Chopped Salad ... 85
- 214 - Carrot & Quinoa Bowl ... 85
- 215 - Seaweed & Carrot Rollups ... 86
- 216 - Middle Eastern Salad ... 86
- 217 - Tropical Tofu Salad ... 87
- 218 - Sweet Broccoli Quinoa Bowl ... 87
- 219 - Cooling Mint Salad ... 88
- 220 - Antioxidant Salad ... 88
- 221 - Minted Quinoa Salad ... 88
- 222 - Sweet & Sour Seaweed Salad ... 89
- 223 - Nutty Snap Pea & Quinoa Salad ... 89
- 224 - Grab & Go Green Wraps ... 90
- 225 - Autumn Salad ... 90
- 226 - Nutty Tacos ... 90
- 227 - Cold Sesame Salad ... 91
- 228 - Tex-Mex Bowl ... 91
... 92

- 229 - Stuffed Eggplant ... 92
- 230 - Chickpea Millet & Cucumber Salad ... 93
- 231 - Sweet Brussel Sprout Salad ... 93
- 232 - Cherry & Fennel Salad ... 93
- 233 - Brussel Sprouts Bowl ... 94
- 234 - Spicy Mexican Salad ... 94
- 235 - Chilled Avocado Soup with Salmon ... 94
- 236 - Asian Pumpkin Salad ... 95
- 237 - Squash & Sprouts Salad ... 95
- 238 - Fennel Citrus Salad ... 95
- 239 - Mushroom Wraps ... 96
- 240 - Sweet Potato Wraps ... 96
- 241 - Refresh Green Grape Salad ... 97
- 242 - Fall Lentil Salad ... 97
- 243 - Brown Rice & Sprouts Salad ... 97
- 244 - Chopped Beet & Quinoa Salad ... 98
- 245 - Sweet Quinoa Salad ... 98
- 246 - Warm Spinach Salad ... 98
- 247 - Veggie Ramen ... 99
- 248 - Spicy Ginger Salad ... 99
- 249 - Curry Squash Soup ... 100
- 250 - Sweet Potato Nacho Boat ... 100
- 251 - Spicy Orange Sweet Potato Bowl ... 101
- 252 - Cauliflower Colcannon ... 101
- 253 - Peas & Rice ... 101
- 254 - Sweet & Spicy Sweet Potato Skillet ... 102
- 255 - Broccoli & Pear Salad ... 102
- 256 - Quinoa Nicoise Salad ... 102
- 257 - Red & Green Salad ... 103
- 258 - Shredded Kale Salad ... 103
- 259 - Italian Kale Stew ... 103
- 260 - Spinach & Beet Salad ... 104
- 261 - Spicy Cabbage Bowl ... 104
- 262 - Fennel Citrus Salad ... 104

DINNER RECIPES ... 105

- 263 - Salmon & Vegetable Kebabs with Greens Pesto ... 105
- 264 - Coconut Curry & Vegetables ... 105
- 265 - Loaded Spaghetti Squash ... 106
- 266 - Asian Noodle Bowl ... 106
- 267 - Spicy Marinara Sauce & Pasta ... 107
- 268 - Lemon Baked Fish Over Green Salad ... 107
- 269 - Cauliflower & Tahini Bowl ... 108
- 270 - Stuffed Peppers ... 108
- 271 - Raw Beetroot Lasagna ... 109
- 272 - Baba Ganoush Pasta ... 109
- 273 - "Cheesy" Broccoli Bowl ... 109
- 274 - Lentil & Green Bean Pesto Salad ... 110
- 275 - Vegetable Packed Minestrone ... 110
- 276 - Noodle Soup with Greens ... 110
- 277 - Southwest Tofu Burger ... 111
- 278 - Zucchini Rolls with Red Sauce ... 111
- 279 - Lentil, Walnut & Arugula Salad ... 112
- 280 - Meatless Taco Wraps ... 112
- 281 - Quinoa & Black Sesame Pilaf ... 113
- 282 - Lemon Zucchini Pasta ... 113
- 283 - Sweet Potato Stew ... 114
- 284 - Cashew Zoodles ... 114
- 285 - Butternut Squash Risotto ... 115
- 286 - Meatless Meatloaf Cups ... 115

287 - Spicy Dal & Greens 116
288 - Blackened Salmon with Fruit Salsa 116
289 - Roasted Cauliflower with Chimichurri Sauce 117
290 - Cook-off Chili 117
291 - Pasta & Veggie Stroganoff 118
292 - Tofu Mole with Jicama Salad 118
293 - Green Pea Pasta 119
294 - Tricolor Pasta 119
295 - Cauliflower Pasta Pillows in Red Sauce 120
296 - Raw Thai Curry 120
297 - Shrimp & Arugula Salad 121
298 - Avocado and Tomato Pizza 121
299 - Spinach Ravioli 122
300 - Kale & Squash Vegetable Gratin 122
301 - Cabbage Rolls 123
302 - Lentil Stuffed Squash 123
303 - Pomegranate Pumpkins 123
304 - Roasted Green Salad 124
305 - Roasted Green Salad 124
306 - Jumbo Stuffed Mushrooms 125
307 - Raw Zoodles with Tropical Sauce 125
308 - Spaghetti Squash Pasta Boats 125
309 - Sweet Potato Chili 126
310 - Sweet Potato Cottage Platter 126
311 - Italian Stuffed Zucchini 127
312 - Sushi Bowl 127
313 - Omega Super Bowl 128
314 - Mediterranean Mushrooms 128
315 - Cauliflower Lettuce Cups 129
316 - Citrus Stir Fry 129
317 - Pineapple Boats 130
318 - Moroccan Vegetable Stew 130
319 - Quinoa Stuffed Peppers 131
320 - Everything Sweet Potato Pizza 131
321 - Lentil Sweet Potato Tacos 132
322 - Spaghetti Squash and Meatless Meatballs 132
323 - Raw Thai Wraps 133
324 - Eggplant & Chickpea Stew 133
325 - Mushroom, Onion & Brown Rice Sauté 134
326 - Tofu Ginger Stir-Fry 134
327 - Cashew Vegetable Skillet 135
328 - Fried Broccoli Rice 135
329 - Coconut Lentil Stew 136
330 - Noodle & Pesto Pizza 136
331 - Farmer's Market Salad 137
332 - Kale Chard Warm Salad 137
333 - Veggie Medley Skillet 137
334 - Indian Onion & Peppers 138
335 - Broccoli Pasta 138
336 - Roasted Vegetable, Hummus & Quinoa Bake 139
337 - Spicy Pepper Soup 139
338 - Rainbow Spaghetti Squash 140
339 - Sweet Tofu & Vegetables 140
340 - Lime Green Pasta 141
341 - Roasted Eggplant & Quinoa 141

DESSERT RECIPES 142
342 - Minted Fruit Salad 142
343 - Apricot Tarts 142
344 - Sweet Potato Tarts 143

345 - Creamy Tropical Ice Pops 143
346 - Nutty Oatmeal Raisin Cookies 144
347 - Raspberry & Chocolate Mousse Jars 144
348 - Refreshing Fruit & Cilantro Pops 144
349 - Lemon Pudding & Raspberry Tarts 145
350 - Coconut Cashew Figs 145
351 - Raw Berry Crumble 146
352 - Coco-nutty Cookies 146
353 - Chocolate Coconut Bites 147
354 - Squash Pudding Parfaits 147
355 - Blueberry Ice Cream 148
356 - Raspberry Cheesecakes 148
357 - Double Chocolate Mint Tarts 148
358 - Brown Rice Pudding 149
359 - Baked Apples with Peanut Butter Sauce 149
360 - Fig Bites 149
361 - Kiwi Lime Squares 150
362 - Chocolate Dipped Apricots 150
363 - Fruit Skewers 150
364 - Mint Chocolate Mousse 151
365 - Raw Chocolate Donut Holes 151
366 - Coconut Raspberry Bites 151
367 - Double Chocolate Cookie Dough Bites 152
368 - Buckwheat Chocolate Crepe Cake 152
369 - Cashew Chip Cookies 152
370 - Pineapple Ice Cream 153
371 - Mixed Fruit Tart 153
372 - Chocolate Orange Cheesecake 154
373 - Summer Crumble 154
374 - Cauliflower Rice Pudding 155
375 - Raw Coconut Lemon Cookies 155
376 - Lemon Lime Jelly Dessert 155
377 - Gingered Pear Bowl 156
378 - Strawberry Coconut Lime Bites 156
379 - Coconut Chip Bites 156
380 - Sweet Potato Orange Cookies 157
381 - Cashew Coconut Cold Cookies 157
382 - Pumpkin Cups 157
383 - Strawberry Roll Ups 158
384 - Pumpkin Pie & Cacao Fudge 158
385 - Strawberry & Lime Balls 158
386 - Papaya Popsicles 158
387 - Lemon Cashew Coated Strawberries 159
388 - Chai Tahini Ice Cream 159
389 - Apricot Crumble 159
390 - Chocolate Sea Salt Popsicles 160
391 - Summer Fruit Mold 160
392 - Baked Pears with Whipped Coconut Cream 160
393 - Mango Mint Mousse Cups 161
394 - Ginger Peach & Raspberry Popsicles 161
395 - Oatmeal Banana Raisin Cookies 161
396 - Raw Mint Chip Cookies 162
397 - Frozen Chocolate Orange Banana Pops 162
398 - Glazed Cinnamon Buns 162
399 - Lemon Sorbet 163
400 - Raspberry Mint Cheesecake Ice Cream 163

Conclusion 164

Introduction

Thank you for taking the time to pick up my book: Alkaline Diet Cookbook - 400 Recipes For Rapid Weight Loss & Maintaining Healthy pH Levels.

This book contains 400 simple, but delicious alkaline recipes that can be consumed on the alkaline diet. The alkaline diet which has become very popular in recent years is a health-based diet that focuses on eating specific foods to make your body more alkaline. Eating more alkaline based foods can help towards individuals trying to lose weight, while it also helps prevent people from developing common life-threatening diseases.

Make sure to keep this cookbook nearby as it's great to come back to when you are in desperate need for a delicious alkaline recipe. With 400 alkaline recipes in this one cookbook, it's going to take you a very long time to make each recipe!

I hope you enjoy this cookbook as much as my other readers have. If you find these alkaline recipes delicious, please leave this cookbook a review on Amazon. Feedback on Amazon really goes a long way and motivates me to keep writing more cookbooks.

BREAKFAST RECIPES

1 - Breakfast Quinoa Salad

Servings: 2
Total Time: 20 minutes

Ingredients:
- 1 teaspoon coconut oil
- ½ cup sweet potato, shredded
- ½ cup of red cabbage, shredded
- ½ cup cooked quinoa
- 2 cups spinach leaves, torn
- 12 cherry tomatoes, halved
- 1 avocado, sliced

Dressing Ingredients

- 1 tablespoon olive oil
- 1 lemon, juiced
- 1 teaspoon Himalayan salt
- ½ teaspoon black pepper
- ½ teaspoon garlic powder

Directions:
1. In a skillet over medium heat, warm coconut oil and add shredded sweet potato and red cabbage. Cook 7 minutes or until slightly softened.
2. Whisk together dressing ingredients in a small bowl.
3. Place quinoa, spinach and cherry tomatoes in a large bowl and pour sweet potato/cabbage mixture over. Stir to combine. Top with avocado and drizzle with dressing.

2 - Carrot & Pineapple Cake Oatmeal

Servings: 2
Total Time: 20 minutes

Ingredients:
- 1 carrot, shredded
- 2 cups water
- 1 cup rolled oats
- ½ pineapple, finely chopped
- ½ teaspoon cinnamon
- ½ teaspoon nutmeg
- ¼ teaspoon ginger powder
- ½ teaspoon vanilla extract
- ¼ cup almond milk
- 2 tablespoons walnuts, chopped
- 2 tablespoons shredded, unsweetened coconut
- 1 tablespoon raisins

Directions:
1. In a saucepan over medium low heat, boil the shredded carrot with the water for 4-8 minutes.
2. Stir in oats, pineapple, cinnamon, nutmeg, ginger and vanilla extract. Simmer over low heat until liquid is gone, and oats are soft, about 6-8 minutes.
3. Stir in almond milk, walnuts, coconut and raisins. Serve warm.

3 - Warming Stew

Servings: 2
Total Time: 20 minutes

Ingredients:
- 2 tablespoons olive oil
- 1 shallot, sliced
- 1 celery stick, diced
- 1 small carrot, diced
- 1 red bell pepper, diced
- 1 garlic clove, minced
- 1 cup green beans, sliced into 1 inch pieces
- 1 cup green cabbage, shredded
- 1 bay leaf
- 2 tablespoons dill, chopped
- 2 tablespoons parsley, chopped
- ½ teaspoon dried oregano
- 3 cups vegetable stock
- 2 cups spinach
- ½ teaspoon sea salt
- ¼ teaspoon black pepper
- 1 cup cooked brown rice

Directions:
1. Heat oil in a large stock pan and add shallot, celery, carrot, red bell pepper and garlic. Let cook 5 minutes or until softened, stirring occasionally.
2. Add green beans and cabbage and cook another 5 minutes or until the cabbage has wilted. Stir in bay leaf, dill, parsley, oregano and then pour in the vegetable stock. Allow to come to a gentle simmer and stir in the spinach. Season with salt and pepper and serve over cooked brown rice.

4 - Sweet Potato Avocado Toasts

Servings: 1
Total Time: 15 minutes

Ingredients:
- 1 small sweet potato, sliced into 1 ½ inch slices
- ½ avocado, mashed
- 1 teaspoon garlic powder
- 1 teaspoon cumin
- ½ teaspoon Himalayan salt
- ½ teaspoon black pepper
- ½ tomato, sliced
- 1 teaspoon sesame seeds

Directions:
1. Place sweet potato slices in toaster and toast on high until slightly browned.
2. In a bowl, mash the avocado, garlic powder, cumin, salt and pepper. Spread on top of sweet potato slices.
3. Place tomato slices on top of the avocado mash and sprinkle with sesame seeds.

5 - Smoky Sweet Potato & Kale Hash

Servings: 2
Total Time: 25 minutes

Ingredients:
- 1 tablespoon coconut oil
- 1 shallot, sliced
- 1 medium sweet potato, diced
- 1 tart apple (such as Granny Smith), cored and diced
- 1 bunch kale (about 14 leaves), de-stemmed and sliced into ribbons
- 1 teaspoon smoked paprika
- ½ teaspoon Himalayan salt
- ¼ teaspoon pepper

Directions:
1. Heat coconut oil in a skillet over medium-low heat. Add shallot and cook 2 minutes or until softened. Add sweet potato and cook 10 minutes being sure to flip potatoes about half way through.
2. Add apple to the pan and cook an additional 2 minutes before tossing in the kale.
3. Season with the paprika, salt and pepper.
4. Cook until kale is slightly wilted and serve warm.

6 - Chopped Breakfast Salad

Servings: 2
Total Time: 10 minutes

Ingredients:
- 1 bunch kale, stems removed and sliced into thin ribbons
- 1 tablespoon olive oil
- 1 teaspoon Himalayan salt
- 1 lime, juiced
- ½ cup quinoa, cooked
- 1 cup watermelon, diced
- ½ cup pineapple, diced
- ½ cup raspberries
- 1 kiwi, diced
- ½ avocado, diced
- 2 tablespoons pepitas

Directions:
1. Place kale in a large bowl and add in the olive oil, salt and 1 tablespoon lime juice. Massage gently and set aside for 5 minutes.
2. After 5 minutes, add quinoa, watermelon, pineapple, raspberries, kiwi, avocado and any remaining lime juice. Toss gently to combine.
3. Sprinkle pepitas on top and serve.

7 - Chai Spiced Breakfast Quinoa

Servings: 1
Total Time: 15 minutes

Ingredients:
- ¼ cup quinoa
- ½ cup water
- ½ cup unsweetened almond milk
- ¼ teaspoon cinnamon
- ¼ teaspoon ground cardamom
- Pinch of ground ginger
- Pinch of ground clove
- 1 tablespoon chia seeds
- 1 teaspoon pepitas
- 1 teaspoon raw honey

Directions:
1. Cook quinoa by combining water, almond milk, quinoa and spices in a medium saucepan over medium heat. Bring to a boil and then reduce the heat to medium and let gently simmer for 5 minutes.
2. Once the water and milk are absorbed and quinoa is light and fluffy, stir in the chia seeds and pepitas. Transfer to a bowl and top with raw honey.

8 - Chia Energy Parfait

Servings: 1
Total Time: 5 minutes

Ingredients:
- ¾ cup unsweetened almond milk
- 3 tablespoons of chia seeds
- ½ teaspoon vanilla extract
- ¼ teaspoon cinnamon
- ¼ teaspoon nutmeg
- 2 tablespoons chopped cashews
- 1 tablespoon unsweetened shredded coconut flakes
- ¼ cup raspberries, slightly mashed
- ¼ cup mango, diced

Directions:
1. Combine almond milk, chia seeds, vanilla, cinnamon, nutmeg and cashews in a glass jar or bowl. Let sit overnight in the fridge.
2. In the morning, layer on top the coconut flakes, raspberries and mango.
3. Serve and enjoy!

9 - Warm Apple Pie Breakfast Cereal

Servings: 2
Total Time: 5 minutes

Ingredients:
- ½ cup quinoa
- 1 ½ cups unsweetened almond milk
- ¼ teaspoon vanilla
- ½ teaspoon cinnamon
- Pinch of allspice
- Pinch of nutmeg
- ½ lemon, juiced
- ¼ cup raisins
- 1 small Granny Smith apple, diced small
- ¼ cup raw almonds, chopped
- 1 teaspoon maple syrup, if desired

Directions:
1. Combine first 9 ingredients in a saucepan over medium heat. Bring to a gentle simmer then reduce heat to low and cook until liquid is absorbed and quinoa is light and fluffy. Transfer to a bowl and top with almonds and maple syrup, if using.

10 - Southwest Tofu Scramble

Servings: 2
Total Time: 15 minutes

Ingredients:
- 1 tablespoon olive oil
- 2 shallots, sliced
- 1 red bell pepper, diced
- 1 cup broccoli florets
- ½ block firm tofu, cubed
- ½ teaspoon cumin
- ½ teaspoon paprika
- ½ teaspoon turmeric
- ¼ cup nutritional yeast
- ¼ teaspoon salt
- ¼ teaspoon pepper
- 3 tablespoons water
- 1 tablespoon cilantro
- 1 avocado, sliced

Directions:
2. Place olive oil in a skillet over medium heat. Add shallots, red bell pepper and broccoli florets. Cook 5 minutes.
3. Add tofu to the pan, breaking up into crumbles with a spoon. Cook another 3 minutes.
4. In a small bowl, mix together cumin, paprika, turmeric, yeast, salt, pepper & water. Pour into the skillet and toss evenly to coat. Cook until liquid evaporates and then stir in cilantro.
5. Transfer to a plate and top with sliced avocado.

11 - Fruity Chia Pots

Servings: 1
Total Time: 5 minutes

Ingredients:
- ¼ cup chia seeds
- 1 cup unsweetened almond milk
- 1 teaspoon vanilla extract
- 1 tablespoon almonds
- 1 tablespoon cashews
- 3 tablespoons fresh blueberries
- 3 tablespoons fresh blackberries
- 2 tablespoons fresh raspberries
- 1 teaspoon raw honey (optional)

Directions:
1. In a medium bowl or jar, combine chia seeds, almond milk and vanilla extract. Once fully combined, let sit overnight in the fridge.
2. The next morning, stir in almonds, cashews, blueberries, blackberries and raspberries. Top with raw honey, if desired.

12 - Sweet Potato Parfait

Servings: 1
Total Time: 35 minutes

Ingredients:
- 1 cup unsweetened plain yogurt
- 1 teaspoon raw honey
- ½ teaspoon fresh ginger, grated
- ¼ teaspoon nutmeg
- ¼ teaspoon cinnamon
- 1 large sweet potato, roasted and flesh removed
- 1 tablespoon walnuts, chopped finely
- 1 tablespoon coconut flakes

Directions:
1. Mix together ¾ cup of yogurt, honey, ginger, nutmeg and cinnamon. Set aside.
2. While still warm, mash the sweet potato flesh lightly.
3. In a deep bowl or jar, add some sweet potato, some yogurt, a few walnuts and coconut flakes. Repeat layers until all ingredients are used up.

13 - Broccoli & Tofu Sandwich

Servings: 2
Total Time: 15 minutes

Ingredients:
- 1 teaspoon coconut oil
- ½ cup broccoli, finely chopped
- 1 shallot, sliced
- ½ block firm tofu
- 1 teaspoon turmeric
- 1 teaspoon dried oregano
- 1 teaspoon garlic powder
- ¼ teaspoon Himalayan salt
- ¼ teaspoon pepper
- 2 tablespoons water
- 3 tablespoons nutritional yeast, divided
- 2 slices sprouted bread, toasted
- 1 avocado, sliced

Directions:
1. In a skillet, heat coconut oil and add broccoli and shallot to sauté. Crumble in tofu and cook 2 minutes.
2. In a small bowl combine turmeric, oregano, garlic, salt, pepper, water and 1 ½ tablespoons of the yeast.
3. Pour spice mixture over the tofu and broccoli mixture. Cook 3 minutes or until liquid is absorbed.
4. Spoon tofu mixture over toasted bread, top with avocado and remaining nutritional yeast.

14 - Nutty Overnight Oats

Servings: 2
Total Time: 10 minutes

Ingredients:
- 1 cup uncooked oats
- 2 cups unsweetened almond milk
- 1 teaspoon vanilla extract
- 1 teaspoon cinnamon
- 1 teaspoon nutmeg
- ¼ teaspoon Himalayan salt
- 2 tablespoons almond butter
- 1 Granny Smith apple, cored and chopped
- 1 tablespoon hemp hearts (optional)

Directions:
1. Mix together oats, almond milk, vanilla, cinnamon, nutmeg and salt. Divide this mixture equally in two jars. Combine mixture well and set in refrigerator overnight.
2. In the morning, add almond butter, chopped apple and hemp hearts to each jar. Serve chilled.

15 - Sunnyside Breakfast Bowl

Servings: 2
Total Time: 20 minutes

Ingredients:
- 1 tablespoon coconut oil
- 1 teaspoon turmeric
- 2 shallots, diced
- 2 garlic cloves, minced
- ½ bunch kale, stems removed and leaves thinly sliced
- ¾ cup yellow split peas, thoroughly rinsed and drained
- 3 cups water
- ½ teaspoon Himalayan salt
- ½ cup grape tomatoes, halved
- 2 scallions, sliced
- 1 avocado, sliced
- 1 sliced breakfast radish
- 2 tablespoons pumpkin seeds, toasted

Directions:
1. In a medium saucepan heat coconut oil over medium heat and add turmeric, shallots, garlic and kale. Cook 5 minutes until kale is wilted. Add split peas and cook for 1 minute.
2. Pour water and salt into the pan, cover and bring to a boil. Reduce heat to low and simmer for approximately 10 minutes.
3. Divide amongst two bowls and top with tomatoes, scallions, avocado, radish and pumpkin seeds.

16 - Turmeric Oats

Servings: 1
Total Time: 20 minutes

Ingredients:
- ½ cup oats
- ¾ cup water
- ¼ cup unsweetened almond milk
- 1 teaspoon turmeric
- 1 teaspoon cinnamon
- ½ teaspoon Himalayan salt
- ¼ teaspoon black pepper, crushed
- 2 tablespoons raisins
- 2 tablespoons coconut flakes, toasted
- 1 tablespoon cacao nibs
- 1/3 cup raspberries

Directions:
1. In a small saucepan over medium-low heat, combine the oats, water, almond milk, turmeric, cinnamon, salt, pepper and raisins.
2. Bring to a boil and then reduce heat to low and simmer until liquid is absorbed.
3. Divide into bowls and top with coconut, cacao and raspberries.

17 - Alkaline Breakfast Raw Mix

Servings: 2
Total Time: 10 minutes

Ingredients:
- ¼ cup almonds, crushed
- ¼ cup pumpkin seeds
- ¼ cup walnuts, crushed
- ½ cup unsweetened coconut flakes
- 1/3 cup rolled oats (gluten-free)
- 2 teaspoons raisins
- 1 teaspoon sesame seeds
- 1 tablespoon raw honey
- 1 ½ tablespoons coconut oil, melted
- 1 teaspoon Himalayan salt
- ¼ teaspoon cinnamon
- ¼ teaspoon nutmeg
- 1 cup unsweetened almond milk
- 1 pear, cored and chopped

Directions:
1. Preheat oven to 300°F/150°C.
2. In a bowl combine the almonds, pumpkin seeds, walnuts, coconut flakes, oats, raisins and sesame seeds.
3. Pour the honey and coconut oil over the mixture and sprinkle with the salt, cinnamon and nutmeg. Toss to combine well and ensure everything is coated.
4. Place mixtures on a parchment lined baking tray and bake for approximately 5 minutes, being careful not to burn.
5. To serve, place mixture in bowls and top with almond milk and pear.

18 - Mexican Breakfast Bowl

Servings: 2
Total Time: 10 minutes

Ingredients:
- 1 ½ cups quinoa, cooked
- 2 tablespoons chia seeds
- 3 tablespoons scallions, thinly sliced
- 1 cup roasted red pepper, diced
- 1 cup cilantro, chopped
- 1 tablespoon nutritional yeast

- 1 teaspoon olive oil
- ½ lime, juiced
- ½ teaspoon Himalayan salt
- ½ teaspoon black pepper, crushed
- ¼ teaspoon cayenne
- ½ cup sprouts

Guacamole
- 1 avocado, pitted and mashed
- 1 shallot, diced
- 1 garlic clove, grated
- ½ lime, juiced

- 1 tablespoon cilantro, chopped
- 1 teaspoon cayenne
- 1 teaspoon cumin
- ½ teaspoon Himalayan salt

Directions:
1. In a large bowl, combine quinoa, chia seeds, scallions, red pepper, cilantro, nutritional yeast, olive oil, lime juice, salt, pepper and cayenne. Mix with a fork to combine well.
2. Make Guacamole by adding all Guacamole ingredients to a small bowl and mixing together.
3. Divide quinoa mixture into two bowls, top each with sprouts and the guacamole.

---

19 - Avocado Zucchini Toast

Servings: 1
Total Time: 10 minutes

Ingredients:
- 2 tablespoons olive oil
- 1 zucchini, grated
- ½ green bell pepper, finely diced
- 1 shallot, finely chopped
- 1 garlic clove, finely minced
- ¼ teaspoon dried oregano
- ¼ teaspoon dried thyme

- ¼ teaspoon dried basil
- ½ teaspoon Himalayan salt
- ½ avocado
- 2 slices gluten-free bread, toasted
- 1 tablespoon pumpkin seeds, toasted
- ¼ cup sprouts

Directions:
1. Heat olive oil in a small skillet over medium heat. Add the zucchini, bell pepper, shallot, garlic, oregano, thyme, basil and salt. Sauté 5 minutes and remove from heat.
2. Mash the avocado and spread over the toast.
3. Top with zucchini mixture, pumpkin seeds and sprouts.

20 - Savory Asian Oatmeal

Servings: 2
Total Time: 15 minutes

Ingredients:
- 1 cup rolled oats
- 2 cups water
- 1 tablespoon olive oil
- 2 tablespoons unsalted peanuts, crushed
- 3 tablespoons green onions, thinly sliced
- ½ jalapeno, seeds removed and diced
- 1 red bell pepper, seeded and diced
- 1 lime, juiced
- 1 teaspoon coconut aminos
- 1 teaspoon tamari
- ⅛ teaspoon chili powder
- ⅛ teaspoon cumin
- ⅛ teaspoon ground cloves
- 1/3 cup cilantro, chopped
- 1 teaspoon peanuts, crushed

Directions:
1. Bring oats and water to boil in a small saucepan over medium heat. Reduce heat to low and simmer about 8 minutes or until liquid is absorbed. Set aside.
2. Heat olive oil in a medium skillet over medium-low heat. Add peanuts, green onions, jalapeno and bell pepper. Sauté 5 minutes or until soft.
3. Stir in lime juice, coconut aminos, tamari and season with chili powder, cumin and cloves.
4. Add oatmeal and cilantro to skillet and stir to combine.
5. Divide into two bowls and top with peanuts.

21 - Breakfast Fruit Crepes

Servings: 2
Total Time: 20 minutes

Ingredients:
- 2 tablespoons ground flax
- 6 tablespoons water
- 1 cup buckwheat flour
- 1 tablespoon coconut oil, melted
- ½ teaspoon Himalayan salt
- ½ teaspoon coconut sugar
- ½ teaspoon vanilla extract
- ¼ teaspoon cinnamon
- 2 cups water
- 2 tablespoons ghee, melted
- 1/3 cup cashew butter
- 2 cups raspberries
- 1 tablespoon cacao nibs

Directions:
1. In a small bowl, whisk together ground flax and water. Place in the fridge for 15 minutes or until a gel is formed.
2. In a blender, combine flax mixture, buckwheat, coconut oil, salt, sugar, vanilla, cinnamon and 2 cups water. Blend well and set aside.
3. Brush ghee on a medium nonstick skillet and place over medium-low heat. Add some of the batter to pan and swirl around entire pan to create even layer. Cook 3 minutes on each side. Remove and repeat until batter is finished.
4. In each crepe, add some of the cashew butter, raspberries and cacao nibs.

22 - Cabbage & Potato Hash

Servings: 2
Total Time: 15 minutes

Ingredients:
- 2 tablespoons olive oil
- 2 small sunchokes, shredded
- 1 cup red cabbage, thinly shredded
- 2 small yellow potatoes, grated
- ¼ cup yellow onion, finely diced
- 1 teaspoon Himalayan salt
- 1 teaspoon rosemary, chopped
- 1 teaspoon black pepper, crushed
- 2 tablespoons green onions, thinly sliced

Directions:
1. Heat oil in a small skillet over medium heat. Add sunchokes, cabbage, potatoes and onion.
2. Cook 10 minutes, stirring frequently.
3. Season with salt, rosemary and pepper. Cook another 5 minutes.
4. Garnish with green onions.

23 - Mediterranean Tofu Scramble

Servings: 2
Total Time: 15 minutes

Ingredients:
- 3 tablespoons olive oil
- 2 cups spinach, chopped
- 1 shallot, thinly sliced
- ½ cup sun dried tomatoes, thinly sliced
- 8 ounces extra firm tofu
- ¼ cup black olives, sliced
- 1 teaspoon oregano
- 1 teaspoon basil
- ½ teaspoon Himalayan salt
- ¼ teaspoon turmeric
- 3 tablespoons water
- 3-4 fresh basil leaves, thinly sliced

Directions:
1. Heat oil in medium skillet over medium-high heat. Add shallot, spinach and sun-dried tomatoes. Cook 5 minutes.
2. Add tofu to the pan and break up with a spoon. Cook 2 minutes and add olives.
3. In a small bowl, combine oregano, basil, salt, turmeric and water. Add to pan and cook 5 minutes or until liquid is evaporated.
4. Garnish with basil leaves.

24 - Tomato Toast

Servings: 2
Total Time: 30 minutes

Ingredients:
- ½ small sweet onion, finely diced
- ½ cup sun dried tomatoes, diced small
- 10 cherry tomatoes, quartered
- 1 garlic clove, grated
- 1 teaspoon oregano
- 1 cup spinach, thinly sliced
- 2 tablespoons olive oil, divided
- 1 tablespoon lemon juice
- 2 teaspoons Himalayan salt
- 1 teaspoon black pepper
- 4 slices sprouted bread, toasted
- 1 tablespoon green onion, thinly sliced

Directions:
1. Preheat oven to 400°F/205°C.
2. On a baking tray lined with parchment paper, combine onion, sun dried tomatoes, cherry tomatoes and garlic. Drizzle with 1 tablespoon olive oil and add oregano and 1 teaspoon of the salt. Toss to coat and make sure mixture is spread evenly over the pan.
3. Place tray in the oven and roast for 25 minutes, flipping once or until tomatoes are soft and slightly caramelized.
4. In a small bowl, combine spinach, remaining olive oil, lemon juice, remaining salt and pepper. Mix well to combine and set aside for 15 minutes.
5. Place spinach mixture on top of toast slices, top with tomatoes and garnish with green onion.

25 - Spicy Tofu Breakfast Bake

Servings: 2
Total Time: 20 minutes

Ingredients:
- 1 teaspoon olive oil
- ½ red onion
- 3 garlic cloves, minced
- 1 green bell pepper
- 1 jalapeno, seeded and diced
- ½ teaspoon smoked paprika
- ½ teaspoon cumin
- 3 tablespoons tomato purée
- 1 cup diced tomatoes
- 2 cups spinach
- 1 teaspoon Himalayan salt
- 8 ounces silken tofu
- 1 tablespoon nutritional yeast
- 2 tablespoons cilantro, chopped

Directions:
1. In a large skillet, heat olive oil over medium-low heat. Add onion, garlic, bell pepper, jalapeno, paprika and cumin. Cook for 5 minutes.
2. Add the tomato purée and diced tomatoes to the pan, reduce heat and let simmer for 10 minutes. Stir in spinach and salt.
3. Add tofu, breaking up gently with a spoon. Sprinkle with nutritional yeast and cook 3 more minutes. Garnish with cilantro and serve.

26 - Coconut Granola

Servings: 2
Total Time: 5 minutes

Ingredients:
- 1 cup oats
- 1/3 cup puffed rice
- ¼ cup walnuts, crushed
- ¼ cup shredded, unsweetened coconut
- 1 tablespoon pumpkin seeds
- ½ teaspoon vanilla extract
- 2 tablespoons raw honey
- 1 teaspoon cinnamon
- 1 teaspoon coconut oil

Directions:
1. Heat oil in a medium skillet over medium-low heat. Add all other ingredients and toss to coat.
2. Cook for 4 minutes, stirring constantly and being sure it does not burn.
3. Transfer to a bowl and let cool before using.

27 - Beet Breakfast Hash

Servings: 2
Total Time: 20 minutes

Ingredients:
- 1 teaspoon olive oil
- 1 onion, diced
- 1 sweet potato, shredded
- 1 large beet, shredded
- 6 ounces firm tofu, cubed
- 6 ounces firm tofu, cubed
- 1 tablespoon coconut aminos
- 1 teaspoon Himalayan salt
- 1 teaspoon black pepper, crushed
- 1 tablespoon parsley, chopped

Directions:
1. Heat olive oil in a medium skillet over medium-high heat. Add onion and cook for 5 minutes before adding the sweet potato and beet.
2. Cook another 10 minutes and then add tofu, coconut aminos, salt and pepper.
3. Sauté another 5 minutes, toss with the parsley and serve.

28 - Citrus Breakfast Salad

Servings: 2
Total Time: 5 minutes

Ingredients:
- 1 persimmon fruit, sliced
- 1 blood orange, sliced into segments
- ¼ cup pomegranate seeds
- 1 tablespoon almonds, toasted and crushed
- ½ cup unsweetened yogurt
- 1 tablespoon lime zest
- 1 teaspoon raw honey

Directions:
1. Toss together persimmon, blood orange, pomegranate seeds and almonds in a medium bowl. Divide mixture amongst two plates.
2. In a small bowl, whisk together the yogurt, lime zest and honey.
3. Top each plate with the yogurt mixture and serve.

29 - Turmeric Citrus Crepes

Servings: 2
Total Time: 30 minutes

Ingredients:
- 1 cup unsweetened almond milk
- 1 egg
- ½ teaspoon vanilla extract
- 1 teaspoon raw honey
- 1 inch piece turmeric, grated
- ½ ginger clove, grated
- ¼ teaspoon cinnamon
- 2 tablespoons lemon zest
- ¾ cup gluten free flour
- 1 teaspoon coconut oil
- 1 cup unsweetened yogurt
- ¼ cup pomegranate seeds

Directions:
1. In a small bowl, whisk together the almond milk, egg, vanilla, honey, turmeric, ginger, cinnamon and lemon zest. Sift in the flour and whisk to combine.
2. Heat coconut oil in a medium skillet over medium-low heat. Pour in a bit of the batter and swirl around the pan, coating the entire bottom. Cook 4-5 minutes then flip and cook another 5 minutes to create the crepes. Set aside and repeat with remaining batter.
3. Divide yogurt and pomegranate amongst each crepe and roll before serving.

---

30 - Sweet Almond Pears

Servings: 2
Total Time: 12 minutes

Ingredients:
- 1 tablespoon coconut oil
- 1 pear, quartered
- ½ cup unsweetened almond milk
- 1 teaspoon vanilla extract
- 1 tablespoon mint, roughly chopped
- ¼ teaspoon cinnamon
- ⅛ teaspoon Himalayan salt
- 1 tablespoon almonds, slivered
- 1 tablespoon raisins

Directions:
1. In a medium saucepan over medium-low heat, heat coconut oil and sear pears on each side until brown, about 3 minutes per side. Remove and set aside.
2. Add almond milk, vanilla, mint, cinnamon and salt to the saucepan. Bring to a low simmer and place pears back in the pan for 3 minutes to soak in the almond milk.
3. Place pears in a serving bowl, pour almond milk on top and top with the almonds and raisins.

---

31 - Berry Oatmeal

Servings: 1
Total Time: 15 minutes

Ingredients:
- ¾ cup unsweetened almond milk
- ¼ cup water
- ½ cup rolled oats
- ¼ teaspoon cinnamon
- ⅛ teaspoon Himalayan salt
- 1 tablespoon almonds, slivered

Berry Jam
- ½ cup raspberries, chopped
- ½ cup frozen blueberries
- 1 lemon, juiced
- ¼ cup chia seeds

Directions:
1. Prepare Berry Jam by placing raspberries, blueberries and lemon juice in a small saucepan over medium heat. Continue stirring the fruit as it cooks, mashing slightly with the spoon. Once berries have melted and thickened, about 3 minutes, stir in the chia seeds and stir well for another 1 minute. Remove and transfer to sealable bowl or jar. You will only use 1 tablespoon of jam for this recipe, but jam can be used throughout the week for other breakfasts or snacks.
2. In a medium saucepan, bring almond milk and water to a rolling boil over medium heat. Stir in the oats, cinnamon, salt and almonds and reduce heat to low. Simmer 3-4 minutes or until liquid is absorbed.
3. Transfer to serving bowl and swirl in 1 tablespoon of the chilled jam. Top with almonds and serve.

32 - Tropical Chia Bowl

Servings: 1
Total Time: 5 minutes plus 8 hours chill time

Ingredients:
- 1 cup chia seeds
- 1 cup unsweetened coconut milk
- ¼ teaspoon vanilla extract
- 1 tablespoon flaxseed, ground
- 1 tablespoon raw honey
- 1 cup pineapple, cubed
- 1 mango, peeled and cubed
- 1/3 cup raspberries
- 1/3 cup coconut flakes, toasted
- ½ tablespoon mint, chopped

Directions:
1. In a medium sized bowl or jar, mix the chia seeds, coconut milk, vanilla extract, flaxseeds and honey. Stir well and let sit (covered) overnight in the fridge.
2. When ready to serve in the morning, add pineapple and mango to a food processor or blender and blend until smooth (add some water if necessary).
3. In your serving bowl, place a layer of the chia mixture and then a layer of the mango/pineapple mixture. Continue layering until both are used up.
4. Top with raspberries, coconut and mint before serving.

33 - Sunshine Granola & Kefir

Servings: 2
Total Time: 1 hour

Ingredients:
- 1 cup gluten-free rolled oats
- 1 tablespoon uncooked quinoa
- 1 tablespoon flaxseeds
- ½ cup walnuts
- ¼ cup pepitas
- 2 tablespoons sesame seeds
- ¼ cup coconut flakes
- 1 orange, zested
- ¼ teaspoon Himalayan salt
- ¼ teaspoon cinnamon
- ¼ teaspoon nutmeg
- 1 tablespoon maple syrup
- 1 tablespoon coconut sugar
- 3 tablespoons coconut oil, melted
- ¼ teaspoon vanilla extract
- 2 cups coconut kefir

Directions:
1. Preheat oven to 350°F/180°C and line a baking tray with parchment paper.
2. In a large bowl, combine the oats, quinoa, flaxseeds, walnuts, pepitas, sesame seeds, coconut flakes, orange zest, salt, cinnamon and nutmeg.
3. In a small bowl, whisk together the maple syrup, coconut sugar, coconut oil and vanilla extract. Pour over the oats and quinoa mixture and toss well to coat. Spread in an even layer on the prepared baking tray. Bake in the oven for 40 minutes, stirring every 10 minutes to prevent burning.
4. Remove, let cool for 10 minutes and serve with coconut kefir.

34 - Sweet Potato & Zucchini Hash Brown

Servings: 2
Total Time: 25 minutes

Ingredients:
- 2 tablespoons flaxseeds, ground
- 6 tablespoons water
- 1 sweet potato, shredded
- 1 zucchini, shredded
- ½ sweet yellow onion, minced
- 2 tablespoons arrowroot
- ¼ teaspoon Himalayan salt
- ¼ teaspoon black pepper, crushed
- 2 tablespoons coconut oil
- 2 tablespoons unsweetened yogurt
- 2 tablespoons chives, sliced

Directions:
1. In a small bowl, whisk together the flaxseeds and water until well combined. Set aside until a gel forms, about 10 minutes.
2. Combine the sweet potato, zucchini, onion, flaxseeds gel, arrowroot, salt and pepper in a medium bowl.
3. Heat coconut oil in a medium sized skillet over medium heat. Form a patty with some of the sweet potato mixture, pressing down slightly and then add it to the skillet. Repeat with remaining sweet potato and zucchini mixture (you may need to make 2 batches depending on your skillet size).
4. Cook 5 minutes or until slightly browned and then flip and cook another 5 minutes.
5. Remove and garnish with the yogurt and chives before serving.

---

35 - Nutty Breakfast Squash

Servings: 2
Total Time: 40 minutes

Ingredients:
- 1 acorn squash, sliced in half lengthwise and seeds removed
- ½ tablespoon coconut oil
- ¼ teaspoon Himalayan salt
- 1 cup unsweetened coconut yogurt, divided
- 4 tablespoons oats
- ½ cup raspberries
- 2 dates, pitted and chopped
- 2 tablespoons cashew butter
- 1 tablespoon raw honey

Directions:
1. Preheat oven to 400°F/205°C and line a baking tray with parchment paper.
2. Rub coconut oil on each cut side of the squash and then sprinkle with salt. Place on the baking tray with cut side down and roast in the oven for 30 minutes or until you can pierce the skin with a fork. Cool for 5 minutes.
3. Take each squash half and fill with half of the yogurt, half of the oats, half the raspberries, 1 date, 1 tablespoon cashew butter and ½ tablespoon honey.
4. Serve immediately.

36 - Spicy Avocado Breakfast Boat

Servings: 2
Total Time: 20 minutes

Ingredients:
- 1 ripe avocado, halved lengthwise and pit removed
- 1 lime, juiced
- 1 tablespoon olive oil
- ½ cup diced red onion
- ½ cup diced red bell pepper
- 1 jalapeno, diced
- 6 ounces firm tofu
- 1 teaspoon nutritional yeast
- ½ teaspoon ground cumin
- ¼ teaspoon oregano
- ⅛ teaspoon ground turmeric
- 1 tablespoon water
- ½ teaspoon black Himalayan salt
- 1 tablespoon fresh chopped cilantro

Directions:
1. Set avocado on two plates and squeeze lime juice on top of each. Set aside.
2. In a medium skillet over medium heat, add olive oil, red onion, bell pepper and jalapeno. Sauté 5 minutes or until onion and pepper are soft.
3. Add tofu to the skillet, breaking up with a spoon and cook 3 minutes.
4. In a small bowl, combine the nutritional yeast, cumin, oregano, turmeric, water and salt. Pour into the skillet and cook 3 more minutes or until the liquid is absorbed.
5. Divide tofu mixture in half and place on top of the avocado half.
6. Garnish with cilantro and serve immediately.

37 - Brussel Sprout Hash

Servings: 2
Total Time: 15 minutes

Ingredients:
- 1 tablespoon olive oil
- 1 shallot, thinly sliced
- 1 sunchoke, sliced thinly
- 4 brussel sprouts, sliced thinly
- ½ sweet potato, shredded
- ½ teaspoon Himalayan salt
- ½ teaspoon black pepper, crushed
- 1 teaspoon fresh rosemary

Directions:
1. Heat olive oil in a medium skillet over medium heat and add the shallot, sunchoke, brussel sprouts and sweet potato.
2. Cook 10 minutes and add salt, pepper and rosemary.
3. Sauté another 5 minutes before removing from heat and serving immediately.

38 - Garden Chickpea Omelet

Servings: 1
Total Time: 25 minutes

Ingredients:
- 1/3 cup chickpea flour
- 2 tablespoons flaxseed, ground
- ½ cup water
- 1 tablespoon lemon juice
- 1 teaspoon tahini
- ½ teaspoon Himalayan salt
- ½ teaspoon black pepper, crushed
- ¼ teaspoon turmeric
- ¼ teaspoon oregano
- ¼ teaspoon garlic powder
- 1 tablespoon olive oil

Filling
- 1 teaspoon olive oil
- 1 small shallot, sliced
- 1 cup spinach
- 5 cherry tomatoes, sliced
- 3 mushrooms, sliced
- ½ avocado, sliced
- 1 tablespoon parsley, chopped

Directions:
1. In a large bowl, thoroughly combine the chickpea flour and flaxseeds. Add in water, lemon juice, tahini, salt, pepper, turmeric, oregano, garlic and whisk to combine. Set aside until mixture is thick, about 5-10 minutes.
2. In a medium skillet over medium-high heat, add teaspoon of olive oil, shallot, spinach, tomatoes and mushrooms. Quickly sauté for 3 minutes until spinach is slightly wilted. Remove and set aside.
3. Add tablespoon of olive oil to the medium skillet and heat over medium heat. Pour chickpea flour mixture into the pan and swirl to ensure it fully covers the bottom of the pan. Let cook for 5-7 minutes and then add the spinach mixture on one side. Fold omelet over and let cook another 2 minutes.
4. Remove from the pan and garnish with parsley before serving.

---

39 - Mocha Pudding

Servings: 1
Total Time: 5 minutes plus 8 hours chill time

Ingredients:
- 1 cup unsweetened almond milk
- ½ teaspoon vanilla extract
- ¼ cup chia seeds
- 2 tablespoons brewed coffee or espresso
- 1 teaspoon raw cacao
- 1 teaspoon cinnamon
- ½ small banana, sliced
- ¼ cup raspberries
- 1 tablespoon raw cacao nibs

Directions:
1. Combine the almond milk, vanilla extract, chia seeds, coffee or espresso, cacao, and cinnamon in a small bowl (that has a cover) or a jar. Stir well to combine, cover and set in the fridge overnight.
2. When ready to eat, top with banana, raspberries and cacao nibs.

40 - Chocolate Chia Breakfast

Servings: 2
Total Time: 20 minutes plus 8 hours chill time

Ingredients:
- 1 ½ cups unsweetened almond milk
- 1 teaspoon dried culinary lavender
- 1 teaspoon earl grey tea leaves
- 1 tablespoon raw honey
- 1 teaspoon vanilla extract
- ¼ cup raw cacao powder
- ¼ cup chia seeds
- 1 tablespoon cacao nibs
- 1 tablespoon walnuts, toasted and crushed

Directions:
1. In a small saucepan over medium heat, add the almond milk, lavender and tea. Let come to a gently boil and then turn heat off and put the lid on to allow lavender and tea to steep for 10 minutes.
2. After milk has sat for 10 minutes, transfer to a medium-sized bowl and add in honey, vanilla and cacao. Stir in the chia seeds, cover and set in the fridge overnight.
3. When ready to eat, top pudding with cacao nibs and toasted walnuts.

41 - Zippy Ginger Breakfast Bars

Servings: 2 (1 bar each)
Total Time: 10 minutes plus 1 hour chill time

Ingredients:
- ¼ cup raw almonds
- ¼ cup raw walnuts
- ½ cup dates, pitted, soaked 10 minutes and then drained
- 1 tablespoon fresh ginger, grated
- ¼ tablespoon cloves
- ¼ teaspoon cardamom
- ¼ teaspoon Himalayan salt

Directions:
1. Add all ingredients to a food processor and mix until a sticky dough forms.
2. Shape dough into two equal sized bars and place on a plate in the fridge for at least 1 hour.

42 - Breakfast Squash Bread

Servings: 2
Total Time: 40 minutes

Ingredients:
- 1 cup almond meal
- 1 tablespoon flax meal
- 1/3 cup arrowroot flour
- ½ tablespoon chia seeds
- ½ teaspoon baking soda
- 1 tablespoon dried oregano
- ½ teaspoon Himalayan salt
- 1 egg
- ½ zucchini, finely grated
- ½ yellow squash, finely grated
- 2 tablespoons coconut milk
- 2 tablespoons coconut oil
- ½ teaspoon apple cider vinegar

Directions:
1. Preheat oven to 350°F/180°C. Line a mini loaf tin with parchment paper.
2. In a medium-sized bowl, combine the almond meal, flax meal, arrowroot, chia seeds, baking soda, oregano and salt.
3. Beat the egg in a large bowl and add the zucchini, squash, coconut milk, coconut oil and vinegar. Pour the dry ingredients into the large bowl with the wet ingredients and stir until well combined.
4. Pour mixture into the prepared mini loaf pan and bake in the oven for 20-30 minutes or until lightly golden brown and cooked in the center.

43 - Cherry Almond Bake

Servings: 2
Total Time: 50 minutes plus 30 minutes cooling

Ingredients:
- 3 tablespoons unsweetened almond milk
- ¼ cup dates, pitted
- 1/3 cup almond meal
- ¾ teaspoon vanilla extract
- ¼ teaspoon almond extract
- ⅛ teaspoon Himalayan salt
- ¼ cup raw almonds, slivered and divided
- 1 ½ cups fresh cherries, pitted, divided
- 1 cup quinoa, cooked

Directions:
1. Preheat oven to 350°F/180°C and line a small baking dish with parchment paper.
2. Combine the almond milk, dates, almond meal, vanilla extract, almond extract, salt, half of the almonds and half of the cherries in a food processor or blender.
3. Add mixture to a large bowl and stir in the quinoa. Pour into prepared baking dish and place remaining cherries and almonds on top.
4. Bake in the oven for 45 minutes or until lightly browned on top.
5. Remove from oven and let cool for 30 minutes before cutting into squares and serving.

44 - Salmon & Cabbage Hash

Servings: 2
Total Time: 12 minutes

Ingredients:
- 1 tablespoon olive oil
- 1 cup green cabbage, thinly shredded
- 1 cup sweet potato, shredded
- 3 green onions, thinly sliced, divided
- 4 ounces smoked salmon, flaked into bite-size pieces
- ¼ teaspoon black pepper, ground
- 1 tablespoon fresh dill, chopped

Directions:
1. In a medium-sized skillet over medium heat, add olive oil, cabbage, sweet potato and half the green onions. Sauté for 8 minutes until cabbage is soft and sweet potato is tender.
2. Add smoked salmon, pepper and dill. Cook 2 minutes.
3. Remove from heat and garnish with remaining green onions before serving.

45 - Summer Medley Parfait

Servings: 2
Total Time: 1o minutes

Ingredients:
- 1/3 cup raw cashews
- ½ tablespoon raw honey
- ½ teaspoon vanilla extract
- ¼ teaspoon almond extract
- 1 teaspoon lemon juice
- ⅛ teaspoon Himalayan salt
- 1 ½ cups strawberries, hulled, chopped and divided
- ½ tablespoon fresh mint, thinly sliced
- 1 cup honeydew, diced
- 1 teaspoon lemon zest
- 1/3 cup almonds, slivered and toasted

Directions:
1. In a food processor, combine the drained cashews, raw honey, vanilla extract, almond extract, lemon juice and salt. Add half of the strawberries and pulse until everything is combined thoroughly.
2. Pour cashew mixture into serving bowls or glasses and top with remaining strawberries, mint, honeydew, lemon zest and almonds.
3. Serve immediately.

46 - Mexican Breakfast Toast

Servings: 2
Total Time: 5 minutes

Ingredients:
- 2 slices sprouted bread, toasted
- 2 tablespoons hummus
- ½ cup spinach, chopped
- ¼ red onion, sliced
- ½ cup sprouts
- 1 avocado, thinly sliced
- ¼ teaspoon Himalayan salt

Spicy Yogurt
- 3 tablespoons unsweetened yogurt
- ½ lime, juiced
- 1 teaspoon cumin
- 1 teaspoon cayenne

Directions:
1. In a small bowl, prepare the Spicy Yogurt by combining all the Spicy Yogurt ingredients and whisking well to combine.
2. Place toast slices on plates and spread a tablespoon of hummus on each. Place spinach on each slice and then Spicy Yogurt, red onion, sprouts and avocado. Sprinkle each with salt and serve.

47 - Omega- Overnight Oats

Servings: 2
Total Time: 5 minutes

Ingredients:
- 1 small ripe banana, mashed
- 1/3 cup rolled oats
- ¾ cup unsweetened almond milk
- ½ teaspoon vanilla extract
- ½ teaspoon cinnamon
- ¼ teaspoon nutmeg
- ⅛ teaspoon Himalayan salt
- 1 tablespoon chia seeds
- 1 tablespoon ground flaxseeds
- 1 teaspoon raw honey
- 1 tablespoon raw almonds, slivered and divided
- ¼ cup blackberries

Directions:
1. Place banana, oats, almond milk, vanilla, cinnamon, nutmeg, salt, chia seeds, flaxseeds, honey and half of the almonds in a medium-sized bowl with a lid or a jar. Stir well to combine and cover.
2. Leave in the fridge overnight.
3. When ready to eat, top with remaining almonds and the blackberries.

48 - Broccoli Omelet

Servings: 2
Total Time: 15 minutes

Ingredients:
- 12 ounces firm tofu
- 3 tablespoons unsweetened almond milk
- 3 tablespoons nutritional yeast
- 3 tablespoons tapioca starch
- 1 teaspoon Dijon mustard
- ¼ teaspoon turmeric
- ¼ teaspoon black pepper, crushed
- 2 tablespoons green onions

Filling
- 1 cup broccoli, steamed
- 1 shallot, sliced
- 2 tablespoons nutritional yeast

Directions:
1. Combine the tofu, almond milk, nutritional yeast, tapioca, mustard, turmeric and pepper in a food processor or blender until smooth.
2. Heat a large, nonstick skillet over medium-high heat until very hot. Pour batter into the skillet and let cook for 7 minutes, being careful not to burn.
3. Place Filling ingredients on one side of the omelet and flip over the other side to cover.
4. Cook another 3 minutes and then transfer to a plate and garnish with green onions.

49 - Tofu & Kale Tacos

Servings: 2
Total Time: 12 minutes

Ingredients:
- 1 tablespoon coconut oil
- 7 ounces extra-firm tofu, drained
- 2 tablespoons nutritional yeast
- 1 teaspoon onion powder
- ¼ teaspoon turmeric
- 1 tablespoon coconut aminos
- 1 cup kale, thinly sliced
- 5 cherry tomatoes, halved
- 4 corn tortillas, warmed
- 1 tablespoon green onions, sliced
- 1 tablespoon cilantro, chopped
- 1 avocado, sliced

Directions:
1. Heat coconut oil in a medium-sized skillet over medium heat. Add tofu, nutritional yeast, onion powder, turmeric and coconut aminos. Cook 5 minutes.
2. Add kale and cherry tomatoes to the skillet and cook another 5 minutes.
3. Remove tofu kale mixture from the stove and divide among the tacos.
4. Top with green onions, cilantro, avocado and serve.

50 - Fruit Porridge

Servings: 2
Total Time: 25 minutes

Ingredients:
- ½ cup whole buckwheat
- ½ cup water
- ½ cup unsweetened almond milk
- 1 tablespoon dried apricot, diced
- 2 tablespoons raisins
- 1 cinnamon stick
- ¼ teaspoon nutmeg
- ¼ teaspoon vanilla extract
- 1 teaspoon ground cardamom
- 1 tablespoon pomegranate seeds
- 1 tablespoon walnuts, toasted and crushed

Directions:
1. In a medium saucepan, add buckwheat, water, almond milk, apricot, raisins, cinnamon, nutmeg, vanilla and cardamom. Bring to a boil and then allow to simmer, stir frequently for 20 minutes or until liquid is absorbed.
2. Remove from heat, remove cinnamon stick and garnish with pomegranate seeds and walnuts before serving.

51 - Morning Sweet Bread

Servings: 2
Total Time: 30 minutes

Ingredients:
- 1 tablespoon flaxseed, ground
- 3 tablespoons water
- 1 ½ cups almond meal
- 2 tablespoons coconut flour
- 1 teaspoon Himalayan salt
- 2 teaspoon cinnamon
- 1 teaspoon vanilla extract
- 1 teaspoon raw honey
- 1 tablespoon olive oil
- 2 tablespoons raisins
- 1 tablespoon cashew butter, melted
- 1 pear, cored and sliced

Directions:
1. Preheat oven to 350°F/180°C and line bottom of a small glass baking dish with parchment paper.
2. In a small bowl, mix together the flaxseeds and 3 tablespoons water to from the flaxseeds gel. Set aside and let sit 10 minutes until it forms a gel.
3. In a large bowl, combine the almond meal, coconut flour, salt, cinnamon, vanilla, honey, flaxseeds gel, olive oil and raisins.
4. Place dough in the baking dish and press into an even layer. Bake in the oven for 15 minutes.
5. Remove and let cool. Top with cashew butter and pear slices before serving.

52 - Banana Breakfast Pudding

Servings: 1
Total Time: 5 minutes plus 8 hours chill time

Ingredients:
- 1 cup coconut milk
- 1 tablespoon raw honey
- ½ teaspoon vanilla extract
- ¼ teaspoon cinnamon
- ¼ teaspoon nutmeg
- ⅛ teaspoon Himalayan salt
- 2 tablespoons chia seeds
- 1 banana, sliced
- 1 tablespoon walnuts, toasted and crushed
- 1 tablespoon cacao nibs

Directions:
1. In a small bowl or jar with a cover, place coconut milk, honey, vanilla, cinnamon, nutmeg, salt and chia seeds.
2. Let sit in the fridge, covered, overnight.
3. In the morning, top with banana, walnuts and cacao nibs before serving.

53 - Italian Breakfast Hash

Servings: 2
Total Time: 35 minutes

Ingredients:
- 2 sweet potatoes, peeled and cubed into ½ inch pieces
- 2 tablespoons olive oil
- ½ red onion, chopped
- ½ red bell pepper, halved and sliced
- ½ green bell pepper, halved and sliced
- 1 garlic clove, minced
- ½ teaspoon Himalayan salt
- ½ teaspoon black pepper, crushed
- ¼ teaspoon paprika
- 4 fresh sage leaves, thinly sliced
- 1 teaspoon oregano
- ¼ teaspoon red chili flakes
- 1 cup tempeh, crumbled
- 1 tablespoon parsley, chopped

Directions:
1. Place sweet potato cubes in a medium pot over medium-high heat. Bring to a boil and let cook 5 minutes. Potatoes should be tender but not mushy. Drain and set aside.
2. Heat oil in a large skillet over medium-low heat. Add onion, both bell peppers, garlic and sweet potatoes. Cook 10 minutes, stirring frequently.
3. Stir in the salt, pepper, paprika, sage, oregano and chili flakes. Cook 2 minutes and then crumble in the tempeh. Cook another 2 minutes and then remove from heat.
4. Garnish with parsley before serving.

54 - Papaya Breakfast Boat

Servings: 2
Total Time: 5 minutes

Ingredients:
- 1 papaya, cut lengthwise in half and seeds removed
- 1 cup unsweetened yogurt
- 1 lime, zested
- 3 tablespoons raw oats
- 1 tablespoon unsweetened shredded coconut
- ½ banana, sliced
- ¼ cup raspberries
- 1 tablespoon walnuts, chopped
- 1 teaspoon chia seeds
- 1 teaspoon raw honey

Directions:
1. Place papaya halves on plates and place yogurt on top of each.
2. Then top each half with lime zest, oats, coconut, banana, raspberries, walnuts, chia seeds.
3. Drizzle with honey and serve.

55 - AM Quinoa Cookies

Servings: 2
Total Time: 25 minutes

Ingredients:
- ¼ cup almond butter
- 1 tablespoon honey
- ½ medium ripe banana, mashed
- 1 egg, beaten
- ½ teaspoon vanilla
- ¼ teaspoon almond extract
- ¼ cup gluten-free oats
- ¼ cup quinoa flakes
- ½ teaspoon baking powder
- ¼ teaspoon Himalayan salt
- ¼ cup unsweetened, shredded coconut flakes, toasted
- 1 tablespoon chia seeds
- 1 teaspoon flaxseed, ground

Directions:
1. Preheat oven to 350°F/180°C and line a baking tray with parchment paper.
2. In a large bowl, combine the almond butter, honey, banana, egg, vanilla and almond extract.
3. In a medium-sized bowl, combine the oats, quinoa flakes, baking powder, salt, coconut flakes, chia seeds and flaxseed.
4. Add the oat mixture to the almond butter mixture and stir well to combine.
5. Using 2 tablespoons as a guide, form small balls and place dough onto the baking tray until all dough is used.
6. Bake in the oven for 15 minutes.
7. Remove and let cool before serving.

56 - Savory Breakfast Bowl

Servings: 1
Total Time: 20 minutes

Ingredients:
- ½ cup rolled oats
- ½ cup unsweetened almond milk
- ½ cup water
- ¼ teaspoon Himalayan salt
- ¼ teaspoon black pepper, crushed
- 1 cup spinach
- 1 tablespoon nutritional yeast
- 1 teaspoon lemon zest
- ½ teaspoon turmeric
- ¼ teaspoon red chili flakes
- 1/3 cup lentils, cooked
- 1 tablespoon green onions, sliced

Directions:
1. In a medium saucepan over medium heat, add oats, almond milk, water, salt and pepper. Bring to a boil and then reduce heat to low and simmer 5-10 minutes or until liquid is absorbed.
2. Stir in the spinach, nutritional yeast, lemon zest, turmeric, chili flakes and lentils.
3. Remove from heat and garnish with green onions before serving.

57 - Almond Butter & Jelly Overnight Oats

Servings: 1
Total Time: 10 minutes plus 8 hours chill time

Ingredients:
- ½ cup rolled oats
- ¾ cup unsweetened almond milk
- ½ teaspoon vanilla extract
- 1 teaspoon chia seeds
- 1 tablespoon almond butter
- 1 tablespoon sliced almonds
- 4 raspberries, sliced

Raspberry Jam
- ¼ cup raspberries, mashed
- 1 teaspoon honey
- 1 tablespoon chia seeds

Directions:
1. In a small bowl, place the ¼ cup mashed raspberries, honey and 1 tablespoon chia seeds. Combine well and set aside in the fridge for 10 minutes.
2. Place oats, almond milk, vanilla, chia seeds and 1 tablespoon of raspberry mixture in a small jar and mix well. Cover and let sit in the fridge overnight.
3. In the morning, add almond butter, sliced almonds and remaining raspberries before serving.

58 - Broccoli & Sprouts Savory Oats

Servings: 1
Total Time: 15 minutes

Ingredients:
- 1 tablespoon olive oil
- 1 shallot, sliced
- 1 teaspoon nutritional yeast
- 1 teaspoon cayenne pepper
- ½ cup rolled oats
- ¾ cup unsweetened almond milk
- ¼ cup water
- 1 cup broccoli florets, steamed and chopped small
- ½ teaspoon Himalayan salt
- ½ teaspoon black pepper, crushed
- ½ cup alfalfa sprouts

Directions:
1. In a medium saucepan over medium heat add the oil, shallot, yeast and cayenne pepper. Cook 5 minutes and then add the oats, almond milk and water.
2. Bring to a boil and reduce heat to low. Cook 5 minutes until liquid is absorbed.
3. Stir in the broccoli, salt and pepper.
4. Remove from heat and top with sprouts before serving.

59 - Fruit & Millet Breakfast

Servings: 2
Total Time: 30 minutes

Ingredients:
- ½ cup millet
- 1 cup water
- 2 tablespoons raisins
- 1 tablespoon currants
- ⅛ teaspoon cinnamon
- ⅛ teaspoon vanilla extract
- 1 cup unsweetened coconut milk, divided
- 1 teaspoon honey
- ½ cup raspberries
- ½ cup blueberries
- 1 teaspoon hemp hearts
- 1 teaspoon chia seeds
- 1 teaspoon mint, chopped

Directions:
1. Place millet and water in a medium saucepan over medium heat. Bring to a boil and then add the raisins, currants, cinnamon and vanilla. Cover with a lid, reduce heat to low and let cook for another 10 minutes until liquid is absorbed.
2. Turn heat off and let sit for 10 minutes
3. Add coconut milk, honey, raspberries, blueberries, hemp hearts and chia seeds. Turn heat to low and let cook for 2 minutes.
4. Transfer to bowls and garnish with mint.

60 - Avocado Breakfast Soup

Servings: 1
Total Time: 5 minutes

Ingredients:
- 1 avocado
- 1 lime, zested and juiced
- ½ cup cucumber, roughly chopped
- ½ cup spinach
- 18 fresh mint leaves
- ⅛ teaspoon Himalayan salt
- 2 tablespoons coconut oil, melted
- 1 tablespoon pepitas
- 1 tablespoon green raisins

Directions:
1. Place all the ingredients, except the pepitas and raisins in a food processor or blender and combine until smooth.
2. Transfer to a bowl and top with pepitas and green raisins.

61 - Sweet Orange Oats

Servings: 2
Total Time: 12 minutes

Ingredients:
- 1 cup sweet potato, cubed, roasted and mashed
- ½ cup oats
- 1/3 cup carrots, grated
- 1 cup unsweetened almond milk
- 2 tablespoons orange juice
- ½ teaspoon ground cinnamon
- ½ teaspoon nutmeg
- ¼ teaspoon Himalayan salt
- 1 teaspoon chia seeds
- ½ persimmon, sliced
- 1 tablespoon orange zest

Directions:
1. In a medium saucepan over medium-low heat, combine mashed sweet potato, oats, carrots, almond milk, orange juice, cinnamon, nutmeg and salt.
2. Bring to a low boil, reduce heat to low and simmer until liquid is absorbed.
3. Stir in chia seeds and garnish with persimmon slices and orange zest to serve.

APPETIZER/SNACKS RECIPES

62 - Greek Zucchini Cups

Servings: 2
Total Time: 10 minutes

Ingredients:
- 2 medium zucchinis, cut into 2 inch pieces and each piece slightly cored to form a cup
- 1 cucumber, finely grated
- 1 cup plain Greek yogurt
- 1 garlic clove, minced
- 1 tablespoon dill, chopped
- 1 tablespoon parsley, chopped
- 1 tablespoon lemon juice
- ½ teaspoon Himalayan salt
- ½ teaspoon black pepper, crushed
- 10 black olives, finely chopped
- 2 tablespoons sprouts

Directions:
1. Prepare zucchini cups and set aside.
2. In a bowl, mix together cucumber, yogurt, garlic, dill, parsley, lemon juice, salt and pepper. Spoon into zucchini cups.
3. Top each cup with some of the olives and sprouts.

63 - Endive & Watercress Boats

Servings: 2
Total Time: 5 minutes

Ingredients:
- 3 cups fresh spinach
- 1 avocado
- 1/2 cup parsley
- ¼ cup mint
- 1 tablespoon lemon juice
- 1 garlic clove
- 1 teaspoon Himalayan salt
- 10 endive leaves
- 1 cup watercress

Directions:
1. Add all ingredients except the endive leaves & watercress to a blender or food processor and blend until smooth, this will form the dip.
2. Scoop dip into each of the endive leaves and top with watercress.

64 - Toasted Trail Mix

Servings: 2
Total Time: 5 minutes

Ingredients:
- 3 tablespoons coconut chips, toasted
- 3 tablespoons walnuts, toasted
- 2 tablespoons almonds, toasted
- 2 tablespoons raisins
- 1 tablespoon pepitas, toasted
- Pinch Himalayan salt

Directions:
1. Combine all ingredients and divide into two equal portions

65 - Chickpea Avocado Cups

Servings: 1
Total Time: 5 minutes

Ingredients:
- 1 very ripe avocado
- ½ cup cooked chickpeas
- ½ tomato, diced
- 1 shallot, diced
- 2 tablespoons olive oil
- 1 tablespoon lemon juice
- ½ teaspoon Himalayan salt
- ½ teaspoon black pepper, crushed
- 1 tablespoon fresh basil, chopped
- 1 teaspoon oregano

Directions:
1. In a small bowl combine chickpeas, tomato, shallot, olive oil, lemon juice, salt and black pepper. Set aside and let rest 5 minutes.
2. Slice the avocado in half lengthwise and remove the pit. Spoon the chickpea and tomato mixture over the middle of each avocado.
3. Garnish with oregano and fresh basil.

66 - Spicy Cocoa-Coco Truffles

Servings: 2
Total Time: 10 minutes

Ingredients:
- 2 cups pitted dates
- ½ cup almond meal
- 1/3 cup shredded unsweetened coconut
- 6 tablespoons raw cacao (or unsweetened cocoa) powder, divided
- ¼ teaspoon sea salt
- ¼ teaspoon cayenne pepper

Directions:
1. Using a food processor on the pulse setting combine the dates, almond meal and shredded coconut until crumbly.
2. Add in 3 tablespoons of the cacao, the sea salt and the cayenne. Blend until the mixture becomes a sticky paste and begins to form a ball.
3. Tear off pieces of the dough and shape into 6 balls. Place remaining cacao on a plate and roll each ball lightly in the cacao.

67 - Adult Ants on a Log

Servings: 1
Total Time: 5 minutes

Ingredients:
- 3 celery stalks, trimmed
- 3 tablespoons almond butter
- 1 tablespoon raisins
- 1 teaspoon sunflower seeds

Directions:
1. Spread almond butter evenly on the celery stalks.
2. Top each piece of celery with raisins and sunflower seeds.

68 - Asian Cucumber Slaw

Servings: 1
Total Time: 15 minutes

Ingredients:
- 1 large cucumber, diced
- 1 garlic clove, minced
- 1 teaspoon fresh ginger, grated
- 2 tablespoons toasted sesame seed oil
- 1 tablespoon brown rice vinegar
- ¼ teaspoon Himalayan salt
- ¼ teaspoon black pepper, crushed
- 1 tablespoon cilantro, chopped

Directions:
1. In a medium bowl, whisk together garlic, ginger, sesame seed oil, vinegar, salt and pepper.
2. Add cucumber and cilantro. Let sit for 5 minutes before serving.

69 - Broiled Grapefruit

Servings: 1
Total Time: 5 minutes

Ingredients:
- ¼ grapefruit
- 1 teaspoon raw honey
- 1 teaspoon almond, crushed
- Pinch flaked sea salt

Directions:
1. Place grapefruit on a broiler pan and broil on high for 3-5 minutes or until lightly brûléed.
2. Spread raw honey on top of the grapefruit and sprinkle with almonds and flaked sea salt.

70 - Coconut Curry Soup

Servings: 2
Total Time: 5 minutes

Ingredients:
- 1 ½ teaspoons coconut oil
- 1 inch piece of ginger, grated
- 2 garlic cloves, minced
- 1 lime, zested
- 1 teaspoon ground coriander
- 1 teaspoon cumin
- ½ teaspoon turmeric
- ½ teaspoon ground mustard
- ½ teaspoon red chili flakes
- ½ teaspoon Himalayan salt
- ¼ teaspoon black pepper, crushed
- 2 small sweet potatoes, peeled and cut into 1 inch pieces
- 1 15 ounce can of full fat coconut milk
- 1 cup filtered water
- ¼ cup cilantro, chopped
- 1 tablespoon pumpkin seeds, toasted
- 2 tablespoons green onions, sliced

Directions:
1. In a large pot over medium heat place coconut oil, ginger, garlic and lime zest. Cook for 5 minutes or until fragrant, being sure to stir frequently.
2. Add coriander, cumin, turmeric, mustard and chili flakes. Continue to stir for another minute before adding in coconut milk, sweet potatoes and water. Bring to a boil then lower heat and simmer for 1 hour.
3. After an hour, turn heat off and let cool completely before adding to a food processor or blender and pureeing until smooth.
4. Place mixture back in the pot and bring to a simmer. Season with salt and pepper.
5. Pour mixture into bowls and garnish with cilantro, pumpkin seeds and green onions.

71 - Chilled Avocado Cilantro Soup

Servings: 2
Total Time: 5 minutes plus 30 minutes chill time

Ingredients:
- 2 cups water
- 1 cup spinach
- 1 avocado, pitted and skin removed
- 1 small cucumber, peeled and seeds removed
- ½ cup cilantro, chopped
- 1 lemon, zested and juiced
- 1 teaspoon Himalayan salt
- ½ teaspoon black pepper, crushed
- ¼ teaspoon cayenne pepper
- 1 inch piece ginger, grated
- 1 garlic clove, grated
- 1 tablespoon cilantro, finely chopped
- 2 tablespoons cucumber, finely diced

Directions:
1. Place all ingredients except for the cilantro and cucumber in a blender and process until smooth to create the soup. Add water if the mixture is too thick.
2. Chill the soup for 30 minutes before garnishing with remaining cilantro and cucumber.

72 - Cooling Cucumber Slice Snack

Servings: 2
Total Time: 5 minutes plus 15 minutes chill time

Ingredients:
- 1 large cucumber, sliced
- 2 garlic cloves, grated
- 1 tablespoon green onion, sliced
- 1 tablespoon toasted sesame oil
- 2 teaspoons apple cider vinegar
- ¼ teaspoon red chili flakes
- ⅛ teaspoon Himalayan salt
- ⅛ teaspoon black pepper, crushed
- 1 teaspoon black sesame seeds

Directions:
1. In a medium bowl whisk together the garlic, green onion, sesame oil, vinegar, chili flakes, salt and pepper.
2. Toss in the cucumber and let sit in the fridge for 15 minutes before sprinkling with sesame seeds and serving.

73 - Spicy Tortilla Soup

Servings: 2
Total Time: 20 minutes

Ingredients:
- 1 tablespoon olive oil
- 1 shallot, diced
- 1 jalapeno, seeded and diced small
- 1 red bell pepper, diced
- 1 tomato, diced
- 1 teaspoon cumin
- 1 teaspoon cayenne pepper
- 1 teaspoon red chili flakes
- 1 cup water
- 1 cup vegetable broth
- ½ cup cilantro, chopped
- 1 cup spinach, chopped
- 1 lime, zested and juiced
- ¼ teaspoon Himalayan salt
- ¼ teaspoon black pepper, crushed
- 1 sprouted tortilla wrap, cut into strips and toasted
- 1 ripe avocado, diced

Directions:
1. In a large pot heat olive oil over medium low heat and add shallot, jalapeno, red bell pepper and tomato for 5 minutes. Add cumin, cayenne and chili flakes and stir for one minute before adding water and vegetable broth.
2. Bring to a boil and then reduce heat and simmer for 15 minutes.
3. Reduce heat and stir in spinach, cilantro, lime zest, lime juice, salt and pepper.
4. Place in bowls and garnish with tortilla strips and avocado.

74 - Raw Green Gazpacho

Servings: 2
Total Time: 5 minutes plus 2 hours chill time

Ingredients:
- 1 medium tomatoes
- 1 green bell pepper, seeds removed and chopped
- 1 tablespoon olive oil
- 1 cup parsley, chopped
- ½ cup cilantro, chopped
- ½ jalapeno, seeded and chopped
- 1 lemon, juiced
- 1 avocado, pitted and flesh removed
- 1 cup vegetable broth
- 1 cup water
- ½ cucumber, diced
- 1 shallot, diced
- 1 tablespoon cilantro, finely chopped
- ½ teaspoon paprika
- ½ teaspoon cumin
- ½ teaspoon cayenne pepper
- ¼ teaspoon Himalayan salt
- ¼ teaspoon black pepper, crushed
- 2 tablespoons green onions

Directions:
1. Add all ingredients except the green onions to a blender and mix until well combined.
2. Chill for 2 hours before garnishing with green onions to serve.

75 - Zesty Green Chips

Servings: 2
Total Time: 5 minutes plus 2 hours chill time

Ingredients:
- 1 bunch kale, stems removed and torn into large pieces
- 1 tablespoon olive oil
- 1 teaspoon Himalayan salt
- 1 teaspoon black pepper, crushed
- 1 teaspoon cayenne pepper
- 1 teaspoon chili powder
- 2 tablespoons nutritional yeast

Directions:
1. Preheat oven to 300°F/150°C and line 2 baking trays with parchment paper.
2. Place kale in a large bowl and pour olive oil on top. Massage kale gently until fully coated.
3. In a small bowl combine salt, pepper, cayenne, chili powder and nutritional yeast. Sprinkle mixture over the kale and make sure every piece is covered with the spice mixture.
4. Lay kale pieces on the baking tray making sure they are in an even layer. Bake 10 minutes, flip pieces over and bake an additional 10 minutes.
5. Remove from oven and let cool.

76 - Mediterranean Spread

Servings: 2
Total Time: 5 minutes plus 2 hours chill time

Ingredients:
- ¼ cup pitted black olives
- ¼ cup pitted green olives
- ¼ cup sundried tomatoes, chopped
- 1 garlic clove, minced
- 1 teaspoon Dijon mustard
- 1 teaspoon fresh thyme leaves, chopped
- 1 teaspoon fresh oregano, chopped
- 2 tablespoons chopped parsley
- ½ lemon, juiced
- 3 tablespoons olive oil
- 1 small Belgian endive, leaves cleaned and trimmed
- Spelt crackers (optional)

Directions:
1. In a food processor combine the black and green olives, tomatoes, garlic, mustard, thyme, oregano and parsley. Scrape down sides and add in lemon juice. Slowly, with the food processor running, drizzle in olive oil.
2. Serve with endive leaves or spelt crackers.

77 - Summer Fruit Soup

Servings: 2
Total Time: 5 minutes plus 1 hour chill time

Ingredients:
- 1 cup cantaloupe, cubed
- 1 cup watermelon, cubed
- 1 cup honeydew, cubed
- 2 tablespoons lime juice
- 1 cup unsweetened coconut milk
- ½ cup water
- 1 tablespoon raw honey
- ⅛ teaspoon Himalayan salt
- 1 tablespoon mint leaves, chopped
- 4 raspberries

Directions:
1. In a food processor combine the cantaloupe, watermelon, honeydew, lime juice, coconut milk, water, honey and salt.
2. Chill 1 hour in the fridge. Garnish with mint and raspberries before serving.

78 - Carrot Tahini Slaw

Servings: 2
Total Time: 15 minutes

Ingredients:
- 1 ½ cups carrots, shredded
- 1 cup red cabbage, shredded
- 1 tablespoon green onions, sliced
- 2 tablespoons raisins
- 3 tablespoons tahini paste
- 1 teaspoon ginger, grated
- 2 teaspoons warm water
- 1 teaspoon lemon juice
- 1 teaspoon raw honey
- ¼ teaspoon Himalayan salt

Directions:
1. In a small bowl whisk together the tahini, ginger, water, lemon juice, honey and salt until smooth. If mixture is too thick, thin out with more water.
2. Mix together the carrots, cabbage, raisins and green onions in a large bowl. Drizzle tahini sauce over vegetables and toss to combine. Let sit for 10 minutes before serving.

---

79 - Veggie Chips

Servings: 2
Total Time: 15 minutes

Ingredients:
- 1 large zucchini, sliced thin
- 1 small beet, peeled and sliced thin
- 1 tablespoon olive oil
- ¼ teaspoon Himalayan salt
- 1 teaspoon garlic powder

Directions:
1. Place zucchini and beet slices on paper towel or tea towel and let sit for 10 minutes to draw out any moisture. Blot slices dry with a fresh towel.
2. Preheat oven to 200°F/95°C and line a baking tray with parchment paper.
3. Place vegetable slices on baking tray in single layer. Brush each side lightly with olive oil and sprinkle with salt and garlic powder.
4. Bake in the oven for 60 minutes or until crispy. Let cool completely.

---

80 - Spiced Middle Eastern Dip

Servings: 2
Total Time: 15 minutes

Ingredients:
- 1 eggplant, sliced into rounds
- ½ teaspoon Himalayan salt
- 1 tablespoon olive oil
- ½ teaspoon olive oil (extra)
- 2 garlic cloves, peeled and grated
- 1 shallot, sliced
- ¼ teaspoon cumin
- ¼ teaspoon red chili flakes
- ⅛ teaspoon black pepper, crushed
- ½ cup parsley, chopped
- 1 tablespoon tahini
- 1 ½ tablespoons lemon juice or more to taste
- ¼ teaspoon Himalayan salt
- 1 cucumber, sliced

Directions:
1. Place eggplant slices on paper or tea towel and sprinkle with ¼ teaspoon salt. Let sit 10 minutes to draw out water. Rinse eggplant and blot dry.
2. Place eggplant slices on a baking tray lined with parchment paper, drizzle with 1 tablespoon olive oil and ¼ teaspoon salt. Roast eggplant in the oven's broiler on high for 5 - 8 minutes or until lightly browned and soft. Remove from oven and peel away the skin.
3. In a food processor, add the eggplant flesh, garlic, shallot, cumin, chili flakes parsley, tahini, lemon juice, remaining ¼ teaspoon salt. Process until well combined.
4. While the food processor is running, drizzle in remaining olive oil. Serve with sliced cucumber.

81 - Detox Soup

Servings: 2
Total Time: 15 minutes

Ingredients:
- 1 ½ beets, peeled and chopped into 1 inch pieces
- 1 stalk celery, chopped
- ½ cup parsley, chopped
- 1/3 cup watercress
- ½ tablespoon coconut oil
- 1 lemon, juiced
- 1 garlic clove, minced
- 2 cups water
- 2 tablespoons apple cider vinegar
- ⅛ teaspoon cayenne pepper

Directions:
1. In a medium saucepan over medium heat, add coconut oil, celery, beets, garlic and lemon juice. Cook 8 minutes until soft.
2. Add water, vinegar and cayenne and bring to a boil.
3. Reduce heat and stir in parsley and watercress. Cook 1 minutes and turn heat off before serving.

82 - Vegetarian Paté

Servings: 2
Total Time: 20 minutes

Ingredients:
- 1 cup green lentils, cooked
- 1 tablespoon olive oil
- ½ cup button mushrooms, sliced
- ½ onion, chopped
- 1 garlic clove, minced
- 2 tablespoons walnuts, toasted
- 1 ½ tablespoons tamari
- ½ cup parsley, chopped
- 1 tablespoon fresh sage, chopped
- ¼ teaspoon black pepper, crushed
- ½ teaspoon Himalayan salt
- 1 teaspoon Dijon mustard
- 1 teaspoon cayenne pepper
- ¼ cup water
- 1 cucumber sliced

Directions:
1. In a medium saucepan over medium-low heat, add olive oil, onions, mushrooms, and garlic. Cook 8 minutes until soft.
2. In a food processor combine the mushroom onion mixture with the cooked green lentils, walnuts, tamari, parsley, sage, pepper, salt, mustard, cayenne pepper and water. Combine until smooth, adding more water if needed. Transfer to a bowl and refrigerate until ready to serve.
3. Serve with cucumber slices

83 - Sage & Butternut Squash Soup

Servings: 2
Total Time: 25 minutes

Ingredients:
- 3 tablespoons olive oil
- 2 shallots, sliced
- 1 garlic clove, minced
- 1 medium butternut squash, peeled and cubed
- 5 fresh sage leaves
- 3 cups vegetable broth
- 1 tablespoon maple syrup
- 1 teaspoon Himalayan salt
- 1 teaspoon black pepper, crushed
- ¼ teaspoon nutmeg
- ¼ cup unsweetened almond milk

Directions:
1. In a medium saucepan over medium-low heat, add 2 tablespoons of olive oil, shallot and garlic and cook 5 minutes until soft. Add in butternut squash, 3 sage leaves, broth, maple syrup, salt, pepper and nutmeg.
2. Bring mixture to a boil, reduce heat and simmer 20 minutes or until squash is soft.
3. When mixture is cooled, add to blender and blend until smooth. Add back to saucepan and bring to a simmer. Pour in almond milk and cook 3 minutes.
4. In a small saucepan over low heat, add 1 tablespoon of oil. When oil is warm, add the 2 unused sage leaves and cook 4 minutes being sure not to burn. Remove sage leaves and set aside.
5. Pour soup into serving bowls and top with frizzled sage leaves.

84 - Chilled Tomato Soup

Servings: 2
Total Time: 10 minutes plus 2 hours chill time

Ingredients:
- 3 tomatoes, peeled
- ½ large green bell pepper, finely chopped
- 1 ½ tablespoons apple cider vinegar
- 1 ½ tablespoons lemon juice
- 1 ½ cucumber, peeled, seeded and finely diced
- 2 shallots, sliced
- 1 jalapeno, seeded and diced
- 1 teaspoon cumin
- 1 teaspoon tamari
- 1 tablespoon olive oil
- 1 ½ tablespoons fresh parsley, chopped
- 1 tablespoon
- 1 teaspoon sugar free hot sauce

Directions:
1. Place all ingredients in a blend and combine until full mixed (mixture will not be entirely smooth). If a thinner soup is desired, add 1 tablespoon of water at a time until desired consistency is achieved.
2. Chill in the fridge for 2 hours before serving.

85 - Sweet & Sour Cabbage

Servings: 2
Total Time: 45 minutes

Ingredients:
- 1 teaspoon ghee
- 1 teaspoon olive oil
- 1 shallot, thinly sliced
- ½ green cabbage, shredded
- ½ red cabbage, shredded
- 2 tablespoons raw honey
- ½ cup apple cider vinegar
- 1/3 cup water
- 1 teaspoon Himalayan salt
- 1 teaspoon black pepper, crushed
- ½ teaspoon nutmeg
- 1 tablespoon caraway seeds

Directions:
1. In a large pot, heat ghee and olive oil over medium heat and add the shallot, green and red cabbage. Cook for 10 minutes or until softened and coated with the oil and ghee.
2. Add honey, vinegar, water, salt, pepper and nutmeg. Cook another 5 minutes then reduce heat to low and simmer for 30 minutes or until cabbage is soft.
3. Stir in caraway seeds and serve warm.

86 - Vegetable & Lentil Soup

Servings: 2
Total Time: 1 hour

Ingredients:
- ½ tablespoon olive oil
- 1 garlic clove, minced
- ¼ cup carrots, diced
- ¼ cup celery, diced
- ¼ cup yellow onion, diced
- 1 small leek, white part sliced into half-moons and cleaned well
- ½ cup brown lentils, washed and drained
- 1 teaspoon dried rosemary
- 1 teaspoon dried thyme
- 2 cups water
- 1 tablespoon tomato paste
- 1 tablespoon apple cider vinegar
- 1 teaspoon Himalayan salt
- 1 teaspoon black pepper, crushed
- Handful spinach leaves

Directions:
1. In a large pot, olive oil and add garlic, onion, carrot, celery and onion. After 5 minutes add the leeks and cook an additional 10 minutes.
2. Add the lentils, rosemary, thyme, water, tomato paste and vinegar. Cook, uncovered, for 45 minutes or until lentils are tender. Stir in spinach leaves and season with salt and pepper before serving.

87 - Roasted Red Pepper Dip

Servings: 2
Total Time: 5 minutes

Ingredients:
- 2 whole roasted peppers
- ¾ cup walnuts, toasted
- ½ cup green onions, sliced
- 2 garlic cloves
- ½ teaspoon Himalayan salt
- 1 tablespoon lemon juice
- 2 teaspoons raw honey
- 1 teaspoon ground cumin
- 1 teaspoon red chili flakes
- ½ teaspoon cayenne pepper
- ½ teaspoon red pepper flakes
- 3 tablespoons almond meal
- 4 tablespoons olive oil

Directions:
1. In a blender or food processor, combine all ingredients except leave a remaining 2 tablespoons of the olive oil.
2. Blend until smooth and transfer to serving bowl. Stir in the remaining 2 tablespoons of olive oil.

88 - Ghee & Maple Roasted Carrots

Servings: 2
Total Time: 35 minutes

Ingredients:
- 3 large carrots, washed and cut into 1 inch pieces
- 1 tablespoon ghee, melted
- 1 tablespoon maple syrup
- 1 teaspoon lemon zest
- 1 teaspoon Himalayan salt
- ¼ teaspoon black pepper, crushed
- 1 tablespoon sesame seeds, toasted

Directions:
1. Preheat oven to 400°F/205°C.
2. In a small bowl, whisk together the ghee, maple syrup, lemon zest, salt and pepper.
3. Place carrots in a shallow baking dish and coat with ghee and maple mixture. Roast 25 minutes, turning once halfway through.
4. Remove carrots from oven and sprinkle the sesame seeds.

89 - Edamame Salad

Servings: 2
Total Time: 20 minutes

Ingredients:
- 1 cup edamame, shelled, cooked and cooled
- 2 tablespoons green onions, sliced
- 1 cup cucumber, diced
- ¼ cup red onion, diced
- 1 teaspoon avocado oil
- 1 teaspoon sesame oil
- ½ teaspoon Himalayan salt
- ¼ teaspoon red chili flakes

Directions:
1. Toss all ingredients in a medium bowl and make sure it is all well coated.
2. Chill in the fridge for 15 minutes before serving.

90 - Smokey Caesar Salad

Servings: 2
Total Time: 15 minutes

Ingredients:
- 1 large bunch kale, stems removes and thinly sliced
- 1 cup pumpkin seeds
- 5 cherry tomatoes, halved
- ½ cucumber, diced
- 1/3 cup almonds
- ⅛ teaspoon chipotle powder
- ½ teaspoon smoked paprika
- 2 garlic cloves
- 1 tablespoon nutritional yeast
- 1 ¼ cup filtered water
- 1 teaspoon honey
- ½ teaspoon Himalayan salt

Directions:
1. In a blender combine the almonds, chipotle powder, smoked paprika, garlic, nutritional yeast, water, honey and salt.
2. Place kale, pumpkin seeds, cherry tomatoes and cucumber in a large bowl and cover with dressing mix from the blender.
3. Toss well to ensure all the leaves are coated and let sit a few minutes before serving.

91 - Baked Sweet Potato Fries with Spicy BBQ Sauce

Servings: 2
Total Time: 35 minutes

Ingredients:
- 1 large sweet potato, cut into large julienne sticks
- 1 tablespoon avocado oil
- ½ teaspoon Himalayan salt
- ½ teaspoon garlic powder

Spicy BBQ Sauce

- 2 tablespoons tomato paste
- 1 tablespoon water
- 1 tablespoon maple syrup
- 1 tablespoon coconut aminos
- 1 teaspoon tamari
- 1 teaspoon smoked paprika
- 1 teaspoon chili powder
- ½ teaspoon cayenne pepper

Directions:
1. Make Spicy BBQ Sauce by combining all the Spicy BBQ Sauce ingredients in a blender.
2. Preheat oven to 400°F/205°C. In a large bowl, toss sweet potato with oil, salt and garlic powder.
3. Place sweet potato on one layer of parchment paper lined on a baking tray. Bake 20 minutes, flipping halfway through.
4. Serve sweet potato fries with the Spicy BBQ Sauce.

92 - Citrus & Jicama Salad

Servings: 2
Total Time: 35 minutes

Ingredients:
- 1 orange, peeled and cut into bite-sized pieces
- 1 grapefruit, peeled and cut into bite sized pieces
- 1 jicama, shredded
- 3 cups spinach
- 3 tablespoons green onions, thinly sliced
- ½ head radicchio, thinly sliced
- 2 tablespoons olive oil
- 2 tablespoons orange juice
- 1 tablespoon lemon juice
- 1 teaspoon lemon zest
- ¼ teaspoon Himalayan salt
- ⅛ teaspoon ground cloves
- ⅛ teaspoon black pepper, crushed

Directions:
1. In a large bowl, combine orange pieces, grapefruit pieces, shredded jicama, spinach, green onions and radicchio.
2. Whisk together the olive oil, orange juice, lemon juice, lemon zest, salt, ground cloves and black pepper in a small bowl to form the dressing.
3. Pour dressing over the citrus and jicama salad and serve.

93 - Green Cabbage Slaw

Servings: 2
Total Time: 15 minutes

Ingredients:
- 1 avocado
- 3 tablespoons olive oil
- 1 lemon, juiced
- 1 teaspoon apple cider vinegar
- ¼ teaspoon Himalayan salt
- ½ cup green cabbage, thinly shredded
- 2 carrots, shredded
- 2 shallots, thinly sliced
- 3 tablespoons cilantro, finely chopped
- 1 tablespoon green onions, thinly sliced
- 1 tablespoon raisins

Directions:
1. Place avocado, olive oil, lemon juice, vinegar and salt in a blender and combine until smooth.
2. In a large bowl combine the avocado mixture, cabbage, carrots, shallots, cilantro, green onion and raisins.
3. Chill 10 minutes before serving.

94 - Spicy Mix with Tortilla Chips

Servings: 2
Total Time: 5 minutes plus 30 minutes chill time

Ingredients:
- 3 tomatoes, finely diced
- 1 green bell pepper, seeded and finely diced
- 2 green onions, thinly sliced
- 2 garlic cloves, grated
- 1 jalapeno, seeded and finely diced
- 2 tablespoons cilantro, finely chopped
- ½ teaspoon Himalayan salt
- ½ teaspoon cayenne pepper
- ¼ teaspoon red chili flakes
- 1 lime, juiced
- 1 tablespoon olive oil
- 24 sprouted corn tortilla chips

Directions:
1. In a medium bowl combine all the ingredients except the tortilla chips. Place half of the mixture in a blender or food processor and pulse 10 times.
2. Add blended mix back to the bowl with the rest of ingredients and stir to combine.
3. Chill at least 30 minutes before serving with tortilla chips.

95 - Creamy Broccoli Soup

Servings: 2
Total Time: 30 minutes

Ingredients:
- 1 small head broccoli, cut into florets
- 1 small avocado
- 1 large shallot, diced
- 1 tablespoon coconut oil
- 1 cup vegetable broth
- ½ cup coconut milk
- 1 teaspoon Himalayan salt
- ½ teaspoon nutmeg
- ½ teaspoon black pepper, crushed

Directions:
1. In a medium saucepan, heat coconut oil over medium high heat. Add shallot and broccoli and cook 10 minutes. Pour in vegetable broth and coconut milk.
2. Bring to a simmer and cook 15 minutes. Let cool and add to blender or food processor along with the avocado and blend until smooth.
3. Add back to saucepan and bring to a simmer. Stir in salt, nutmeg and black pepper.

96 - Chilled Coconut Soup

Servings: 2
Total Time: 5 minutes plus 3 hours chill time

Ingredients:
- 1 small head cauliflower, steamed or roasted
- 1 cup unsweetened coconut milk
- 1 cup water
- 2 tablespoons lime juice
- 2 tablespoons coconut oil
- 1 tablespoon cream of coconut
- 2 teaspoons cilantro, chopped

Directions:
1. Add cauliflower, coconut milk, water, lime juice, coconut oil and cream of coconut in a food processor. Blend until smooth, adding more water if it is too thick.
2. Transfer to a large bowl and chill 2-3 hours. Garnish with cilantro before serving.

97 - Root Vegetable Soup

Servings: 2
Total Time: 35 minutes

Ingredients:
- 2 tablespoons coconut oil
- 2 medium shallots, sliced
- 1 inch piece ginger, peeled and sliced
- 4 carrots, chopped
- 1 sweet potato, peeled and chopped
- 2 parsnips, chopped
- 3 cups vegetable stock
- 1 teaspoon Himalayan salt
- 1 teaspoon black pepper, crushed
- ¼ teaspoon cinnamon
- ⅛ teaspoon nutmeg

Directions:
1. Heat oil over medium heat in a medium saucepan. Add shallots and ginger and cook 5 minutes. Add carrots, sweet potato and parsnips. Cook another 10 minutes, stirring frequently.
2. In the saucepan, add the vegetable stock and bring to a boil. Reduce heat and simmer for 20 minutes or until vegetables are soft.
3. Let mixture cool before adding to a blender and mixing until smooth. If using an immersion blender, skip cooling the mixture.
4. Transfer back to saucepan and bring to a simmer over low heat. Stir in salt, pepper, cinnamon and nutmeg.

98 - Squash Dip with Cucumber Slices

Servings: 2
Total Time: 5 minutes

Ingredients:
- 1 cup pumpkin puree
- 1 avocado, pitted and flesh removed
- ½ red bell pepper, chopped
- 2 green onions, chopped
- 1 teaspoon cumin
- 1 teaspoon coriander
- 1 teaspoon ground cardamom
- ½ teaspoon turmeric
- ½ teaspoon cinnamon
- 1 tablespoon lemon juice
- 1 teaspoon Himalayan salt
- 1 teaspoon black pepper, crushed
- 1/3 cup water
- 1 cucumber, sliced

Directions:
1. Add all the ingredients except the cucumber to a high speed blender and combine until smooth to create the dip.
2. Serve with cucumber slices.

99 - Creamy Two Bean Salad

Servings: 2
Total Time: 10 minutes

Ingredients:
- 1 cup white beans
- 1 cup celery, chopped
- ½ cup fresh green beans, chopped into 1 inch pieces
- ½ cup chopped organic red onion, or green onion
- 1 cup watercress
- 1 apple, chopped

Dressing
- 2 inch piece of fresh ginger peeled and sliced thin across the grain
- 2 tablespoons coconut oil
- 1 lime, juiced
- 1 tablespoon raw honey
- 1 teaspoon Himalayan salt
- 1 cup coconut milk
- ½ cup coconut cream
- 1 teaspoon, black pepper

Directions:
1. Combine white beans, celery, green beans, onion, watercress and apple in a large bowl.
2. In a blender combine Dressing ingredients until smooth.
3. Pour Dressing over bean mixture and toss to coat.
4. Serve immediately.

---

100 - Chilled Beet Soup

Servings: 2
Total Time: 30 minutes

Ingredients:
- 1 tablespoon coconut oil
- 1/3 cup yellow onion, diced
- 1 cup beets, peeled and chopped
- 1/3 cup carrots, shredded
- 1 cup red cabbage, shredded
- 2 cups vegetable broth
- 1 teaspoon Himalayan salt
- 1 teaspoon black pepper, crushed
- 1 tablespoon fresh dill, chopped
- ½ cup unsweetened coconut milk

Directions:
1. In a large saucepan over medium heat, add the coconut oil, onion, beets and carrots. Cook 10 minutes before adding the cabbage.
2. Cook an additional 5 minutes and add vegetable broth, salt, pepper and dill. Reduce heat to low and simmer for 15 minutes.
3. Using an immersion blender, blend mixture until smooth. Stir in coconut milk, transfer to a bowl and allow to sit for 5 minutes before serving.

---

101 - Green Hummus

Servings: 2
Total Time: 5 minutes

Ingredients:
- 1 garlic clove
- 2 tablespoons green onion, sliced
- 1 cup chickpeas, drained and rinsed
- 2 tablespoons lemon juice
- ½ cup parsley, chopped
- 1 cup spinach, chopped
- 1 tablespoon cup tahini
- 2 tablespoons olive oil
- 2 tablespoons water
- 1 teaspoon cumin
- 1 teaspoon cayenne pepper
- ½ teaspoon Himalayan salt
- ¼ teaspoon black pepper
- 2 carrot, cut into sticks
- 2 celery stalks, trimmed and cut in half

Directions:
1. In a food processor or blender, combine all ingredients except the carrots and celery to create the hummus. Add more water if mixture is too thick.
2. Transfer to a small bowl and serve with carrots and celery.

102 - Spinach Artichoke Dip

Servings: 2
Total Time: 5 minutes

Ingredients:
- 1 14 ounce can of artichoke hearts
- 2 cups spinach, chopped
- 1 15 ounce can of chickpeas
- 2 tablespoons parsley, chopped
- 4 tablespoons olive oil
- 1 lemon, juiced
- 2 garlic cloves, minced
- 4 tablespoons nutritional yeast
- 1 teaspoon chili powder
- 1 teaspoon paprika
- 1 teaspoon Himalayan salt
- 1 teaspoon black pepper, crushed
- 2 carrot, cut into sticks
- 2 celery stalks, trimmed and cut in half

Directions:
1. Combine all ingredients except the carrots and celery in a food processor or blender and combine until well combined (but still able to see pieces of artichoke and spinach) to create the dip.
2. Serve with carrots and celery.

103 - Spinach Cabbage Soup

Servings: 2
Total Time: 30 minutes

Ingredients:
- 1 tablespoon olive oil
- ¼ cup red onion, diced
- 1 garlic clove, minced
- 1 celery stalk, diced
- 1 medium carrot, diced
- ½ cup mushrooms
- ½ head of broccoli, cut into florets
- ½ cup red bell pepper, diced
- 1 teaspoon fresh ginger, peeled and minced
- ½ turmeric
- ⅛ teaspoon cayenne pepper
- 1 teaspoon Himalayan salt
- 1 teaspoon black pepper, crushed
- 3 ½ cups vegetable broth
- 2 cups spinach, roughly chopped
- ½ cup purple cabbage, thinly shredded
- ¼ cup parsley, chopped

Directions:
1. In a large pot, heat olive oil over medium heat. Add onion, garlic, celery and carrot. Cook 5 minutes and then add mushrooms, broccoli, pepper and ginger. Cook an additional 10 minutes.
2. Sprinkle vegetables with turmeric, cayenne, salt and pepper. Cook for 1 minute and add vegetable broth.
3. Bring to a boil then reduce heat and simmer 10 minutes.
4. Stir in spinach, cabbage and parsley, cook another minute and then serve immediately.

104 - Fermented Greens

Servings: 2
Total Time: 30 minutes (plus 3 days of fermenting)

Ingredients:
- 1 cup cabbage, thinly sliced
- 1 cup kale, stems removed and thinly sliced
- 1 cup cucumber, diced
- ½ cup carrot, shredded
- 2 tablespoons green onions, thinly sliced
- 2 tablespoons Himalayan salt
- 1 garlic clove, grated
- 1 tablespoon ginger, grated
- 1 teaspoon cayenne pepper
- 1 tablespoon red chili flakes
- 1 tablespoon smoked paprika
- 2 cups water

Directions:
1. In a large bowl combine the cabbage, kale, cucumber, carrot and green onion. Add salt and massage for 5 minutes, making sure to squeeze vegetables during the 5 minutes.
2. In a sterilized jar with a lid, add the vegetable mix with the remaining ingredients.
3. Place jar on a counter in a cool, shaded area for at least 3 days.
4. Put in fridge after 3 days and chill for a few hours before serving.

105 - Coconut Asparagus Soup

Servings: 2
Total Time: 20 minutes

Ingredients:
- 1 tablespoon coconut oil
- 1 shallot, sliced
- 1 garlic clove, minced
- 1 tablespoon green curry paste
- 1 15 ounce can coconut milk
- 1 cup water
- 2 cups asparagus, trimmed and chopped into 1 inch pieces
- 1 cup baby spinach, chopped
- 1 teaspoon Himalayan salt
- 1 teaspoon black pepper, crushed
- 1 tablespoon lime juice
- 1 tablespoon green onions, sliced
- 1 tablespoon cilantro, chopped

Directions:
1. In a large saucepan over medium heat add coconut oil, shallot and garlic. Cook 3 minutes and then add the curry paste. Cook an additional 1 minute.
2. Pour in the coconut milk, water and asparagus. Bring to a boil and then reduce heat to low and simmer for 15 minutes.
3. Stir in spinach, salt and pepper. Using an immersion blender, blend mixture until smooth. Stir in lime juice.
4. Garnish with green onion and cilantro.

106 - Vegetable & Rice Stew

Servings: 2
Total Time: 20 minutes

Ingredients:
- 1 teaspoon olive oil
- 1 green onion, thinly sliced
- 1 garlic clove, minced
- 1 carrot, sliced into coins
- 1 celery stalk, sliced
- 1 cup white mushrooms, sliced
- ½ cup leeks, sliced
- ¼ cup brown rice
- 2 cups baby kale
- 3 cups vegetable broth
- 1 teaspoon Himalayan salt
- 1 teaspoon black pepper, crushed
- 1 teaspoon dried oregano
- ¼ teaspoon red chili flakes
- ¼ cup fresh parsley, chopped

Directions:
1. Heat olive oil in a large saucepan over medium heat. Add onion, garlic, carrot, celery, mushrooms and leeks. Cook 10 minutes.
2. Stir in rice and kale and cook 1 minute before adding vegetable broth. Let it come to a boil then reduce heat to low and simmer 15 minutes.
3. Season with salt, pepper, oregano and chili flakes.
4. Before serving, stir in parsley.

107 - Dairy Free Fruity Milk Jar

Servings: 1
Total Time: 15 minutes

Ingredients:
- ½ cup raspberries
- 1 teaspoon mint, chopped
- 1 teaspoon raw honey
- ¼ cup chia seeds
- 1 cup unsweetened almond milk

Directions:
1. In a medium sized jar, add raspberries, mint and honey. Mash with the handle of a wooden spoon.
2. Add chia seeds and almond milk and stir to combine.
3. Let sit for 10 minutes before serving.

108 - Cleansing Soup

Servings: 2
Total Time: 25 minutes

Ingredients:
- 1 tablespoon avocado oil
- 1 shallot, sliced
- 2 garlic cloves, sliced
- 1 inch ginger, sliced
- ½ teaspoon ground cumin
- ¼ teaspoon ground turmeric
- 1 ½ cups zucchini, zucchini
- 1 cup broccoli, florets trimmed
- 1 cup spinach
- ½ cup green bell pepper, seeds removed and chopped
- 3 cups water
- 1 teaspoon Himalayan salt
- 1 lemon, zested and juiced
- 2 tablespoons parsley

Directions:
1. Heat oil over medium heat in a large saucepan. Add shallot, garlic, ginger, cumin, turmeric and cook for 5 minutes. Add in zucchini, broccoli, spinach and bell pepper.
2. Cook another 8 minutes before stirring in the water, salt and lemon juice. Let cook another 5 minutes or until the vegetables are tender.
3. Place vegetable mixture in a blender or food processor and add the lemon zest and parsley. Blend until smooth and serve warm.

109 - Red Citrus Salad

Servings: 2
Total Time: 10 minutes

Ingredients:
- 1 tablespoon cup coconut aminos
- ¼ cup apple cider vinegar
- 3 tablespoons orange zest
- 2 tablespoons orange juice
- 1 tablespoon maple syrup
- 1 tablespoon olive oil
- 1 teaspoon Himalayan salt
- 3 cups spinach
- ½ radicchio, thinly shredded
- 3 cups beets, peeled, chopped and roasted
- 1 cup red onion, diced
- 1 cup pomegranate seeds
- 2 tablespoons walnuts, toasted and crushed

Directions:
1. In a small bowl, whisk together the coconut aminos, vinegar, orange zest, orange juice, maple syrup, olive oil and salt.
2. In a large salad bowl, toss together the spinach, radicchio, beets, red onion, and pomegranate seeds. Drizzle with dressing and toss to coat. Garnish with walnuts.

110 - Sweet Summer Soup

Servings: 2
Total Time: 15 minutes

Ingredients:
- 1 medium honeydew melon
- 2 tablespoons lemon juice
- ¼ cup fresh raspberries
- ¼ cup fresh strawberry
- ½ cucumber, peeled and diced
- ¼ cup coconut milk (from a can)

Directions:
1. Place all ingredients, except the coconut milk in a blender and mix until smooth.
2. Pour into serving bowls and pour coconut milk into each as garnish.

111 - Melon Pie

Servings: 2
Total Time: 15 minutes

Ingredients:
- 4 circular slices of a small watermelon
- 1/3 cup unsweetened yogurt
- 3 kiwis, sliced
- ½ cup strawberries, sliced
- ¼ cup blueberries
- 10 grapes, halved
- ¼ teaspoon cinnamon
- 1 teaspoon raw honey
- 2 teaspoons mint leaves, chopped

Directions:
1. Lay out watermelon slices and spread yogurt on each slice.
2. Top with kiwi, strawberries, blueberries and grapes. Sprinkle cinnamon on each slice.
3. Drizzle with honey and top each slice with mint leaves.

112 - Super Smooth Parsnip Soup

Servings: 2
Total Time: 30 minutes

Ingredients:
- ½ tablespoon olive oil
- 2 shallots, sliced
- 1 celery stalk, chopped
- 1 garlic clove, crushed
- 1 teaspoon fennel seeds
- 1 parsnip, chopped
- ¼ teaspoon cayenne pepper
- 2 cups vegetable stock
- ½ medium cauliflower head, cut into florets
- ½ teaspoon Himalayan salt
- ½ teaspoon black pepper, crushed
- 1 tablespoon green onions, sliced

Directions:
1. In a large saucepan over medium heat, add oil, shallots, celery, garlic and fennel seeds. Cook for 5 minutes or until softened. Add in parsnips and cayenne pepper. Cook 2 minutes.
2. Add vegetable stock, cauliflower, salt and pepper. Bring to a low boil then reduce heat to low and simmer 15 minutes.
3. Blend cooled soup in a blender or food processor until smooth. Reheat in a saucepan over medium heat. Ladle into bowl, garnish with green onions and serve.

113 - Cucumber & Salmon Cups

Servings: 2
Total Time: 10 minutes

Ingredients:
- 1 large cucumber, sliced into 1 ½ inch slices
- 10 - 12 smoked salmon pieces
- 10 - 12 dill fronds
- ½ tablespoon olive oil
- ½ teaspoon black pepper, crushed

Directions:
1. For each cucumber slice, hollow out one end so that you can create a little cup.
2. Fold the smoked salmon piece enough so that you can fit it in the cucumber cup hole. Add a dill frond to each cup.
3. Drizzle with olive oil and sprinkle with black pepper.

114 - Sweet Potato Toasts

Servings: 2
Total Time: 15 minutes

Ingredients:
- 1 small sweet potato, sliced into 1 ½ inch slices
- ½ cup raspberries
- ½ lime, juiced
- 1 teaspoon lime zest
- 1 tablespoon chia seeds
- 3 tablespoons cashew butter
- 1 tablespoon pumpkin seeds, toasted
- 1 tablespoon raisins

Directions:
1. Place sweet potato slices in griller and grill/toast on high until slightly browned.
2. In a small bowl, mash the raspberries along with the lime juice and zest. Stir in chia seeds and let sit for 10 minutes.
3. Spread cashew butter on each slice of sweet potato. Then add the raspberry chia jam spread you created on each slice.
4. Top with pumpkin seeds and raisins.

115 - Eggplant Cashew Bites

Servings: 2
Total Time: 15 minutes

Ingredients:
- 1 eggplant, very thinly sliced
- 1 tablespoon olive oil
- 1 teaspoon Himalayan salt
- 1 tablespoon pine nuts
- 1 tablespoon raisins

Cashew Basil Filling
- 1 cup cashews, soaked overnight and drained
- 1 lemon, juiced
- 3 tablespoons water
- 1 tablespoon nutritional yeast
- ½ teaspoon Himalayan salt
- ¼ teaspoon ground nutmeg
- 1 handful fresh basil, roughly chopped

Directions:
1. Place broiler on high and line a baking tray with parchment paper.
2. Brush each slice of eggplant with olive oil and season with salt. Place on the baking tray. Broil 4 minutes and then flip to broil 4 minutes on the other side.
3. Make Cashew Basil Filling by placing all ingredients in a food processor and blending until smooth.
4. Remove Cashew Basil Filling from food processor and mix in the pine nuts and raisins.
5. Place Cashew Basil Filling in each of the eggplant slices and roll up, securing with a toothpick.

116 - Curry Chips

Servings: 2
Total Time: 35 minutes

Ingredients:

- 1 bunch curly kale, stems removed and torn into pieces

Curry Spice Mix
- 1 tablespoon melted coconut oil
- 1 tablespoon lemon juice
- 2 garlic cloves, minced
- 1 teaspoon turmeric
- 1 teaspoon red chili flakes
- 1 teaspoon Himalayan salt
- ½ teaspoon black pepper, crushed
- ¼ teaspoon ground ginger
- ¼ teaspoon coriander
- ¼ teaspoon cardamom
- ⅛ teaspoon cumin

Directions:
1. In a small bowl, combine the coconut oil, lemon juice, garlic, turmeric, chili flakes, salt, pepper, ginger, coriander, cardamom and cumin.
2. Line two baking trays with parchment paper and preheat oven to 275°F/135°C.
3. Pour Curry Spice Mix over all the kale and toss well to coat, ensuring spices get into every part of the kale leaves. Place kale on baking tray and place in the oven.
4. Bake the kale chips for 30 minutes, rotating pans once.

117 - Mexican Dip

Servings: 2
Total Time: 30 minutes

Ingredients:
- 1 cup lentils, cooked
- 1 garlic clove, minced
- ½ teaspoon cumin
- ½ teaspoon Himalayan salt
- 2 tablespoons green onions, sliced

Salsa
- 1 tomato, diced
- ½ green bell pepper
- ½ red onion, diced
- ½ lime, squeezed
- 1 tablespoon cilantro, chopped

Yogurt
- 1 cup unsweetened goat yogurt
- ½ teaspoon cumin
- ½ teaspoon cayenne pepper

Guacamole
- 1 avocado
- 1 garlic clove, grated
- 1 jalapeno, seeded and diced
- ½ red onion, diced
- ½ teaspoon Himalayan salt

Directions:
1. Make base layer by combining lentils, 1 garlic clove, ½ teaspoon cumin and ½ teaspoon salt in a small bowl. Spread on the bottom of a small glass baking dish. Make salsa layer by combining the all the salsa ingredients together in a bowl. Place this mixture on top of the lentils.
2. Using another bowl, whip together the yogurt ingredients and place on top of the salsa.
3. In a small bowl, mash together the guacamole ingredients to make the guacamole. Spread on top of the yogurt layer.
4. Garnish with green onions and serve with cut up vegetables.

118 - Three Onion Soup

Servings: 2
Total Time: 45 minutes

Ingredients:
- 2 tablespoons ghee
- 1 large yellow onion, peeled and thinly sliced
- 1 large leek, sliced
- ¼ cup green onions, sliced
- 3 small potatoes, quartered
- 2 garlic cloves, minced
- 3 cups vegetable broth
- 1 teaspoon Himalayan salt
- 1 teaspoon black pepper, crushed

Directions:
1. In a large stockpot over medium heat, add ghee, yellow onions, leeks and green onions. Cook 10-15 minutes, lightly caramelizing the onions.
2. Add potatoes, garlic and broth. Bring to a boil and then reduce heat to low and simmer 25 minutes or until potatoes are tender.
3. Season with salt and pepper before serving.

119 - Watermelon, Mint & Tofu Kebabs

Servings: 2
Total Time: 10 minutes

Ingredients:
- 8 watermelon cubes
- 8 tofu cubes
- 8 mint leaves
- 1 tablespoon olive oil
- 1 teaspoon Himalayan salt
- 1 teaspoon black pepper, crushed
- 4 bamboo skewers, cut in half

Directions:
1. On each skewer, place a watermelon cube, tofu cube and a mint leaf.
2. Drizzle each skewer with olive oil and sprinkle with salt and pepper

120 - Blackberry Salsa

Servings: 2
Total Time: 15 minutes

Ingredients:
- 1 teaspoon avocado oil
- 1 tablespoon raw honey
- 3 tablespoons lime juice
- 1 tablespoon lime zest
- 1 cup blackberries
- 1/3 cup green onions, chopped
- 1 cup chopped fresh cilantro
- 1 jalapeno, seeded and diced
- ¼ cup pumpkin seeds, toasted
- ¼ teaspoon Himalayan salt

Directions:
1. Whisk together the avocado oil, honey, lime juice and lime zest in a small bowl.
2. In a large bowl, muddle the blackberries gently with the end of a spoon. Add in green onions, cilantro, jalapeno and pumpkin seeds.
3. Pour oil and honey mixture over the blackberries. Season with salt and toss to combine.
4. Chill 10 minutes before serving with cut up vegetables.

121 - Smokey Nut Mix

Servings: 2
Total Time: 10 minutes

Ingredients:
- 1 teaspoon coconut oil
- 2 tablespoons honey
- 1 tablespoon coconut aminos
- ½ cup pecans
- ½ cup almonds
- ½ teaspoon cinnamon
- ¼ teaspoon cayenne pepper
- ⅛ teaspoon smoked paprika

Directions:
1. In a small bowl, combine all the ingredients and make sure the nuts are well coated.
2. Preheat oven to 300°F/150°C and line a baking tray with parchment paper.
3. Spread nuts on the baking tray and ensure they are in a single layer.
4. Place baking tray in the oven and cook for 5 minutes, stirring frequently to ensure they do not burn.
5. Remove and let cool in a small bowl.

122 - Seaweed Spread

Servings: 2
Total Time: 10 minutes

Ingredients:
- 1 cup cashews, soaked overnight and drained
- 1 teaspoon dried dulse seaweed
- 1 teaspoon dried wakame
- 1 garlic clove, minced
- 1 teaspoon black pepper, crushed
- ½ lemon, juiced
- ½ teaspoon dill, chopped
- ½ teaspoon Himalayan salt
- 1 tablespoon apple cider vinegar
- ¼ cucumber, chopped
- 4 teaspoons red onion, minced
- ½ cup celery, minced

Directions:
1. Blend the first 9 ingredients together in a food processor until smooth but still with some texture.
2. Transfer to medium sized bowl and fold in the cucumber, red onion and celery.
3. Serve with cut up vegetables or gluten-free crackers.

123 - Spring Soup

Servings: 2
Total Time: 35 minutes

Ingredients:
- 1 tablespoon olive oil
- 2 shallots, sliced
- 1 cup asparagus, trimmed and cut into 1-inch pieces
- ½ cup artichoke hearts
- 1 garlic clove, minced
- 1 ½ cups vegetable broth
- ¼ cup water
- 1 teaspoon apple cider vinegar
- ½ teaspoon oregano
- ¼ teaspoon turmeric
- ¼ teaspoon cayenne pepper
- ½ teaspoon Himalayan salt
- ½ teaspoon black pepper, crushed
- ½ lemon, juiced
- 1 tablespoon chives

Directions:
1. In a medium saucepan over medium heat, add oil, shallots, asparagus, artichoke and garlic. Cook 8 minutes and then add the broth, water, vinegar, oregano, turmeric, cayenne, salt and pepper.
2. Bring to a boil and then reduce heat to low and simmer 15 minutes.
3. Let cool slightly and transfer to a food processor or blender. Blend until mixture is smooth.
4. Place back in the saucepan over medium-low heat and bring to a simmer before stirring in lemon juice.
5. Garnish with chives before serving.

124 - Herbed Mushrooms

Servings: 2 (5 mushrooms each)
Total Time: 20 minutes

Ingredients:
- 1 cup cashews, soaked 3 hours then drained and rinsed
- 1 garlic clove, chopped
- 1 tablespoon lemon juice
- ½ teaspoon Himalayan salt
- ½ cup silken tofu
- 1 tablespoon nutritional yeast
- ¼ teaspoon cayenne pepper
- ¼ cup fresh dill, chopped
- ¼ cup fresh parsley, chopped
- ¼ teaspoon black pepper, crushed
- 10 mushrooms, stems removed
- 5 cherry tomatoes, halved

Directions:
1. Preheat oven to 350°F/180°C. Line a baking tray with parchment paper.
2. Place cashews, garlic, lemon juice, salt and tofu in a food processor and blend until well combined and smooth.
3. Add nutritional yeast, cayenne, dill, parsley and pepper to the food processor and blend until incorporated.
4. Stuff each mushroom with the cashew mixture and top with half a tomato.
5. Bake in the oven for 15 minutes or until mushrooms are soft.
6. Serve immediately.

125 - Guacamole Hummus

Servings: 2
Total Time: 5 minutes

Ingredients:
- 2 avocados
- 2 cups of chickpeas, cooked
- 1 tablespoon tahini
- 1 garlic clove, minced
- 3 tablespoons lemon juice
- ½ teaspoon cumin
- ½ teaspoon red chili flakes
- 1 tablespoon avocado oil
- ½ teaspoon Himalayan salt
- ¼ teaspoon black pepper, crushed
- 2 tablespoons cilantro, chopped
- 1 cucumber, sliced
- 1 carrot, cut into sticks

Directions:
1. Combine all ingredients, except cucumber and carrots, in a food processor until smooth.
2. Serve with cucumbers and carrots

126 - Avocado & Tomato Salad

Servings: 2
Total Time: 5 minutes

Ingredients:
- 2 avocados, diced
- 4 Roma tomatoes, quartered
- ¼ cup red onion, thinly sliced
- 2 tablespoons cilantro
- ½ teaspoon Himalayan salt
- ½ teaspoon black pepper, crushed

Directions:
1. Combine all ingredients in a medium-sized bowl and toss well.
2. Serve immediately either on its own or with some crackers.

---

127 - Cheesy Zucchini Chips

Servings: 2
Total Time: 5 minutes plus 2 hours bake time

Ingredients:
- 1 large zucchini, sliced thinly
- 2 tablespoons olive oil
- 1 teaspoon Himalayan salt
- 2 teaspoons onion powder
- 1 teaspoon garlic powder
- 2 tablespoons nutritional yeast

Directions:
1. Preheat oven to 200°F/95°C. Line a baking tray with a parchment paper.
2. Toss all ingredients in a large bowl so that the zucchini is evenly coated.
3. Place on baking tray and bake for 2 hours or until crispy.

---

128 - Curry Pepper Hummus

Servings: 2
Total Time: 5 minutes plus 2 hours bake time

Ingredients:
- 1 red bell pepper
- 2 tablespoons olive oil
- ½ cup chickpeas
- 1 tablespoon tahini
- 1 garlic clove
- ½ lemon, juiced
- ½ teaspoon Himalayan salt
- ½ teaspoon curry powder
- ¼ teaspoon turmeric
- ¼ teaspoon chili flakes
- 1 teaspoon cilantro
- 1 cucumber, sliced
- 1 carrot, cut into sticks

Directions:
1. Place all ingredients except the cilantro, cucumber and carrot into a food processor and blend until smooth.
2. Garnish with cilantro and serve with cucumber and carrot.

129 - Mushroom & Onion Kebabs

Servings: 2
Total Time: 35 minutes

Ingredients:
- 2 tablespoons olive oil
- 1 garlic clove, minced
- 1-inch piece ginger, grated
- ½ tablespoon tamari
- ½ tablespoon coconut aminos
- 1 teaspoon lime juice
- 1 teaspoon lime zest
- ½ tablespoon red chili flakes
- 15 cremini mushrooms, stems removed and sliced
- ½ red onion, quartered
- ½ teaspoon Himalayan salt
- 4 bamboo skewers, soaked 15 minutes
- 1 tablespoon cilantro, chopped

Directions:
1. Place olive oil, garlic, ginger, tamari, coconut aminos, lime juice, lime zest and red chili flakes in a medium bowl. Whisk together well and add mushrooms, onion and salt.
2. Let mushrooms and onions sit for 15 minutes and then place on the skewers in alternating pattern.
3. Heat a grill pan over medium-high heat and grill mushroom skewers for 5 minutes on each side.
4. Garnish with cilantro and serve immediately.

130 - Open Faced Avocado Sandwich

Servings: 2
Total Time: 5 minutes

Ingredients:
- 2 slices sprouted bread, toasted
- 2 tablespoons hummus, divided
- 1 ripe avocado, sliced and divided
- 4 tomato slices
- 4 cucumber slices
- 1 tablespoon sunflower seeds
- 1 teaspoon nutritional yeast
- ½ teaspoon Himalayan salt
- ½ teaspoon black pepper, crushed

Directions:
1. Top each slice of toast with hummus, avocado, 2 tomato slices, 2 cucumber slices, sunflower seeds, nutritional yeast, salt and pepper.
2. Serve immediately.

131 - Mediterranean Parsnip Fries

Servings: 2
Total Time: 25 minutes

Ingredients:
- 5 parsnips, cut into strips or wedges
- 2 tablespoons olive oil
- 2 garlic cloves, minced
- 1 teaspoon dried oregano
- 1 teaspoon dried thyme
- 1 teaspoon dried basil
- 1 teaspoon onion powder

Directions:
1. Preheat oven to 400°F/205°C. Line a baking tray with parchment paper.
2. Add all the ingredients to a medium-sized bowl and toss well to coat.
3. Lay parsnips on a baking tray in an even layer.
4. Bake in the oven for 20 minutes or until crispy.

132 - Spicy Sweet Potato Bites

Servings: 2
Total Time: 30 minutes

Ingredients:
- 1 small and narrow sweet potato, sliced into thin slices
- 1 teaspoon olive oil
- ½ teaspoon cayenne pepper
- ¼ teaspoon smoked paprika
- ¼ teaspoon garlic powder
- ¼ teaspoon Himalayan salt
- 1 avocado, mashed
- ¼ cup tomato, diced
- 1 garlic clove, minced
- 1 shallot, diced
- ½ lime, juiced
- 1 tablespoon cilantro, chopped

Directions:
1. Preheat oven to 400°F/205°C. Line a baking tray with parchment paper.
2. Add the sweet potato, olive oil, cayenne, paprika, garlic powder and salt to a medium-sized bowl and toss well to coat.
3. Lay sweet potatoes on baking tray in an even layer. Bake in the oven for 20 minutes or until crispy.
4. While sweet potatoes are in the oven, combine the avocado, tomato, garlic, shallot, lime and cilantro in a medium-sized bowl until well combined.
5. Remove sweet potatoes from the oven and let cool for 5 minutes.
6. Top with avocado mixture and serve.

133 - Scallion Chickpea Cakes

Servings: 2
Total Time: 20 minutes

Ingredients:
- ¾ cup chickpea flour
- ½ cup water
- ¼ teaspoon garlic powder
- ½ teaspoon Himalayan salt
- ½ teaspoon black pepper, crushed
- 2 shallots, diced
- ½ cup green onion, sliced
- 2 tablespoons, cilantro
- 1 tablespoon coconut oil
- 2 tablespoons tamari
- 1 tablespoon coconut aminos
- 1 teaspoon chives, chopped

Directions:
1. Combine all the ingredients, except the coconut oil, tamari, coconut aminos and chives in a medium-sized mixing bowl and stir until combined to form the batter.
2. Heat coconut oil in a medium skillet over medium-high heat. Add two tablespoons of batter to the skillet in a circular shape. Let cook 4-5 minutes or until browned on the bottom and flip.
3. Cook another 4 minutes and then remove.
4. Combine the tamari and coconut aminos in a small dish.
5. Garnish the cakes with the chives and serve with tamari sauce.

134 - Sweet Chili Carrot Fries

Servings: 2
Total Time: 30 minutes

Ingredients:
- 8 large carrots, cut into wedges
- 1 tablespoon avocado oil
- 1 teaspoon garlic powder
- ½ teaspoon Himalayan salt
- ½ teaspoon cayenne pepper
- ¼ teaspoon coconut sugar

Chili Sauce

- 2 tablespoons coconut aminos
- 1 tablespoon honey
- 1 teaspoon red chili flakes

Directions:
1. Preheat oven to 400°F/205°C. Line a baking tray with parchment paper.
2. Place carrots, oil, garlic, salt, cayenne and coconut sugar in a large mixing bowl and toss well to coat.
3. Lay carrots on a baking tray in an even layer and bake in the oven for 25 minutes or until crispy.
4. While carrots bake, mix together the Chili Sauce ingredients in a small bowl.
5. Remove carrots and serve with Chili Sauce.

135 - Spiced Apple Slices

Servings: 2
Total Time: 5 minutes

Ingredients:
- 1 red apple, core removed and sliced into circular slices
- ½ teaspoon lemon juice
- 3 tablespoons cashew butter
- 1 tablespoon raisins
- 1 tablespoon sunflower seeds
- ½ teaspoon cinnamon powder

Directions:
1. Place apple slices on a plate and drizzle with the lemon juice (to prevent browning).
2. Spread cashew butter on each of the apple slices and then top with raisins, sunflower seeds and cinnamon powder.
3. Serve immediately.

136 - Coconut Butter Dates

Servings: 2
Total Time: 5 minutes

Ingredients:
- 10 dates, pitted
- 2 tablespoons coconut butter

Directions:
1. Stuff each date with some of the coconut butter.
2. Chill 10 minutes before serving.

137 - Warm Avocado Cups

Servings: 2
Total Time: 8 minutes

Ingredients:
- 1 ripe avocado, pitted
- 1 teaspoon coconut oil
- ¼ teaspoon cayenne pepper
- 2 tablespoons honey
- 1 tablespoon coconut aminos
- ¼ cup pepitas, toasted
- 1 tablespoon cilantro, chopped

Directions:
1. Brush coconut oil on each open side of the avocado and then sprinkle with cayenne.
2. Heat grill pan over medium-high heat and add avocado, keep the cut side facing down. Cook 5 minutes or until lightly grilled.
3. Remove avocados from pan, drizzle with honey and coconut aminos and then top with pepitas and cilantro.

138 - Fruit Salsa

Servings: 2
Total Time: 25 minutes

Ingredients:
- ½ pineapple, finely chopped
- ½ cucumber, finely chopped
- ½ mango, finely chopped
- ½ green bell pepper, finely chopped
- ¼ cup green onion, sliced
- 2 limes, zested and juiced
- 1/3 cup cilantro, roughly chopped
- 1 teaspoon cayenne pepper
- ½ teaspoon Himalayan salt
- ½ teaspoon coconut aminos
- 1 cup sprouted tortilla chips or crackers

Directions:
1. Combine all ingredients, except the chips in a medium mixing bowl.
2. Let sit in the fridge for 20 minutes before serving with tortilla chips.

139 - Chocolate Orange Pineapple Rings

Servings: 2
Total Time: 10 minutes plus 30 minutes chill time

Ingredients:
- ¼ cup coconut oil
- 2 tablespoons cacao powder
- 1 tablespoon maple syrup
- 10 dried pineapple rings
- 1 tablespoon unsweetened, shredded coconut
- 1 teaspoon almonds, slivered
- 1 teaspoon cacao nibs
- 1 teaspoon orange zest
- ¼ teaspoon Himalayan salt

Directions:
1. In a small bowl, combine coconut oil, cacao and maple syrup to create the chocolate mixture.
2. Line a baking tray with parchment paper.
3. Dip half of a pineapple ring in chocolate mixture. Lay on baking tray and sprinkle with some of the coconut, almonds, cacao nibs, orange zest and salt (sprinkle on the chocolate side).
4. Repeat with remaining pineapple rings and toppings.
5. Chill 30 minutes in the fridge before serving.

140 - Raspberry Mint Yogurt Pops

Servings: 2
Total Time: 5 minutes plus 2 hours chill time

Ingredients:
- 1 teaspoon honey
- 2 cups unsweetened yogurt
- ¼ cup mint, finely chopped
- ½ cup raspberries

Directions:
1. In a small bowl, combine the honey, yogurt and mint.
2. Place a few raspberries in the bottom of 4 popsicle molds. Add in some of the yogurt mixture and then add a few more raspberries. Top each mold with remaining yogurt mixture.
3. Place in the freezer for at least 2 hours.

141 - Cheesy Bean Chips

Servings: 2
Total Time: 35 minutes

Ingredients:
- 3 cups green beans
- ¼ cup avocado oil
- 2 teaspoon Himalayan salt
- ¼ cup nutritional yeast
- 1 teaspoon garlic powder
- 1 teaspoon onion powder
- 1 teaspoon paprika
- ½ teaspoon cayenne pepper

Directions:
1. Preheat oven to 400°F/205°C. Line a baking tray with parchment paper.
2. Toss all ingredients in a medium-sized bowl to properly coat the green beans.
3. Place green beans on the baking tray and bake in the oven 30 minutes or until crispy.

142 - Banana Strawberry Bites

Servings: 2
Total Time: 10 minutes plus 1 hour freeze time

Ingredients:
- 2 large bananas, sliced into ½ inch pieces
- 1/3 cup almond butter
- 3 strawberries, sliced
- 3 tablespoons coconut oil, melted
- 1 tablespoon raw cacao powder
- 1 teaspoon maple syrup
- ¼ teaspoon Himalayan salt

Directions:
1. Take a banana slice and spread each slice with some almond butter. Top with a strawberry slice and then put a banana slice on top to make a sandwich.
2. In a small bowl, combine the oil, cacao, maple syrup and salt to form the chocolate mixture.
3. Dip each banana sandwich in the chocolate mixture and place on a parchment paper lined baking tray.
4. Freeze at least 1 hour in the freezer before serving.

143 - Spinach & Artichoke Stuffed Mushroom

Servings: 2
Total Time: 20 minutes

Ingredients:
- 6 white button mushrooms, stems removed and chopped (keep the remaining head of the mushroom)
- 1 cup spinach, steamed and chopped
- ¼ cup canned artichoke, drained and chopped
- ¼ cup nutritional yeast
- 1 tablespoon olive oil
- ¼ teaspoon garlic powder
- ¼ teaspoon onion
- ⅛ teaspoon pepper
- ¼ teaspoon Himalayan salt

Directions:
1. Add the mushroom stems, spinach, artichoke, nutritional yeast, olive oil, garlic, onion, pepper and salt to a food processor. Pulse a few times until combined but not entirely smooth.
2. Preheat oven to 350°F/180°C and line a baking tray with parchment paper.
3. Stuff each mushroom head with the spinach and artichoke mixture and place on the parchment paper.
4. Bake for 15 minutes.
5. Remove and serve hot.

144 - Quick Avocado Wraps

Servings: 2
Total Time: 5 minutes

Ingredients:
- 4 Romaine lettuce leaves
- 1 avocado, sliced
- 1 ½ cups sprouts
- ½ cup hummus
- 1 cucumber, sliced
- 1 tablespoon sunflower seeds
- ¼ teaspoon Himalayan salt
- ¼ teaspoon black pepper, crushed

Directions:
1. Stuff each lettuce leaf with the avocado, sprouts, hummus, cucumber, sunflower seeds, salt and pepper.
2. Roll up and enjoy.

145 - Strawberry Toast

Servings: 2
Total Time: 5 minutes

Ingredients:
- 2 slices sprouted bread, toasted
- 3 tablespoons almond butter
- 2 tablespoons unsweetened yogurt
- 4 strawberries, hulled and sliced
- ½ teaspoon cinnamon
- 1 tablespoon chia seeds
- 1 tablespoon sunflower seeds

Directions:
1. Spread almond butter on each of the slices of toast.
2. Top with yogurt, sliced strawberries, cinnamon, chia seeds and sunflower seeds.
3. Serve immediately.

146 - Triple Berry Parfait

Servings: 2
Total Time: 5 minutes

Ingredients:
- ½ cup strawberries, hulled, sliced and divided
- ½ cup raspberries, divided
- ½ cup blueberries, divided
- 1 tablespoon chia seeds
- 1 ½ cups unsweetened yogurt
- 2 tablespoons mint, chopped
- 3 tablespoons almonds, slivered

Directions:
1. Layer strawberries in the bottom of two tall glasses. Top with half the chia seeds and then a quarter of the yogurt.
2. Top with half raspberries and a half the almonds.
3. Top with half blueberries and half mint.
4. Repeat with remaining glass and ingredients.

147 - Sweet & Savory Almonds

Servings: 2
Total Time: 30 minutes

Ingredients:
- 1 cup raw almonds
- 2 tablespoons raw honey
- 1 tablespoon coconut aminos
- 1 tablespoon tamari
- ½ tablespoon garlic powder
- ½ tablespoon onion powder
- ½ teaspoon celery salt

Directions:
1. Preheat oven to 350°F/180°C. Line baking tray with parchment paper.
2. Toss all the ingredients in a medium bowl until well coated.
3. Place almonds on baking tray in an even layer.
4. Bake in the oven for 25 minutes, stirring every 5 minutes so almonds don't burn.

148 - Plantain Chips

Servings: 2
Total Time: 25 minutes

Ingredients:
- 2 large green plantains, sliced
- 1 tablespoon coconut oil
- ½ tablespoon Himalayan salt
- ¼ teaspoon onion powder

Directions:
1. Preheat oven to 350°F/180°C. Line baking tray with parchment paper.
2. Toss all the ingredients in a medium-sized bowl until well coated.
3. Add plantain slices to baking tray and bake in the oven for 20 minutes, flipping once after 10 minutes until they are cooked properly to create the "plantain chips."
4. Remove and let cool before serving.

149 - Coconut Figgy Toast

Servings: 2
Total Time: 5 minutes

Ingredients:
- 2 sliced sprouted bread, toasted
- 2 tablespoons coconut butter
- 3 fresh figs, sliced
- 1 tablespoon unsweetened, shredded coconut
- 1 teaspoon chia seeds

Directions:
1. Spread coconut butter on top of cooled toast slices. Place figs on top of each slice.
2. Sprinkle with shredded coconut and chia seeds.

150 - Tamari Pepitas Snack

Servings: 2
Total Time: 25 minutes

Ingredients:
- ½ cup pepitas
- 2 tablespoons tamari
- ½ teaspoon coconut aminos
- 1 teaspoon garlic powder
- ½ teaspoon cayenne pepper

Directions:
1. Preheat oven to 350°F/180°C. Line baking tray with parchment paper.
2. Toss all the ingredients in a medium-sized bowl until well coated.
3. Add pepitas to baking tray and bake in the oven for 20 minutes, stirring every 5 minutes
4. Remove and let cool before serving. Great to keep in a ziplock bag and snack on throughout the day.

151 - Sweet Roasted Chickpeas

Servings: 2
Total Time: 35 minutes

Ingredients:
- 2 cups chickpeas, cooked
- 1 tablespoon coconut oil
- 1 teaspoon cinnamon
- 1 teaspoon nutmeg
- 1 teaspoon coconut sugar

Directions:
1. Preheat oven to 400°F/205°C. Toss chickpeas with coconut oil in a small oven proof bowl. Bake in the oven for 30 minutes, mixing frequently.
2. While chickpeas bake, add cinnamon, nutmeg and sugar to a separate medium sized bowl.
3. Remove chickpeas from oven and place immediately in the bowl with the spices. Toss well to coat.
4. Lay on a plate and let cool before serving.

152 - Roasted Broccoli with Tahini Dip

Servings: 2
Total Time: 35 minutes

Ingredients:
- 2 cups broccoli, cut into large florets
- 2 tablespoons olive oil
- ½ teaspoon Himalayan salt
- ¼ teaspoon turmeric
- 2 tablespoons tahini
- 1 tablespoon warm water
- ½ tablespoon honey

Directions:
1. Preheat oven to 400°F/205°C. Toss broccoli with oil, salt and turmeric in a small oven proof bowl. Bake in the oven for 30 minutes, turning once.
2. While broccoli roasts, whisk together the tahini, water, and honey in a small bowl.
3. Remove broccoli from oven and serve immediately with the tahini dip.

DRINK RECIPES

153 - Green Goddess Smoothie

Servings: 1
Total Time: 5 minutes

Ingredients:
- 1 avocado
- ½ cucumber
- 1 cup of fresh kale leaves, stems removed
- 1 peeled lime
- ½ cup chopped parsley
- 1 cup water

Directions:
1. Place all ingredients into a high speed blender. Pulse a few times to get started then mix on high until smooth.

154 - Spicy & Smooth Green Shake

Servings: 2
Total Time: 5 minutes

Ingredients:
- 1 cucumber
- 2 tomatoes
- 1 avocado
- 1 cup spinach leaves
- 1 lime, juiced
- ½ jalapeno, seeded
- ¼ teaspoon red pepper flakes
- ½ cup water
- 1 teaspoon spirulina powder

Directions:
1. Combine all ingredients in a blender and combine until smooth. Add more if too thick.

155 - Tropical Smoothie

Servings: 2
Total Time: 5 minutes

Ingredients:
- 1 cup pineapple, diced
- 1 cup watermelon, diced
- 2 limes, juiced
- ½ cup cauliflower florets, steamed
- ½ cup cilantro, chopped
- ½ cup coconut water

Directions:
1. Place all ingredients in a blender and blend until smooth.

156 - Ginger Blast Smoothie

Servings: 2
Total Time: 5 minutes

Ingredients:
- 2 cucumbers, roughly chopped
- 1 lemon, juiced
- 1 lime, juiced
- 2 inch piece of ginger, peeled and sliced
- 2 cups spinach
- 1 apple, cored and roughly chopped
- 1 cup water
- 2 teaspoons chia seeds

Directions:
1. Place all ingredients except the chia seeds in a blender and blend until smooth. Stir in chia seeds and serve.

157 - Spicy Golden Tea

Servings: 2
Total Time: 10 minutes

Ingredients:
- 16 ounces water
- 1 inch of fresh turmeric root, peeled and diced small
- 1 inch of fresh ginger root, peeled and diced small
- 2 lemon slices (do not boil, add to tea before serving)
- 2 teaspoons raw honey
- Pinch black pepper

Directions:
1. Place water, turmeric and ginger in a small saucepan and bring to a boil over medium heat.
2. Reduce heat and let simmer another 5 minutes.
3. Pour into glasses and add lemon slices, honey and pepper before serving.

158 - Lemon Basil Zinger

Servings: 2
Total Time: 5 minutes

Ingredients:
- 2 small lemons, peeled and seeds removed
- 1 ½ tablespoons of coconut oil
- ½ green apple, cored and chopped
- 3 ½ cups water
- ½ teaspoon Himalayan salt
- 1 teaspoon raw honey
- 3 fresh basil leaves
- 4 - 5 ice cubes
- 2 lemon slices

Directions:
1. Place all ingredients in a blender except the lemon slices and blend until fully combined.
2. Serve with a fresh lemon slice.

159 - Bloody Mary Shake

Servings: 2
Total Time: 10 minutes

Ingredients:
- 1 small cucumber
- 1 celery stalk
- 3 tomatoes
- ½ red bell pepper, seeded and roughly chopped
- 1 garlic clove
- 1 lemon, juiced
- ½ jalapeno, seeded
- ¼ teaspoon pepper
- ½ teaspoon tamari sauce
- ¼ teaspoon cayenne pepper
- 6 - 8 ice cubes
- 4 olives

Directions:
1. Place all ingredients in a blender except for the olives and blend until fully combined.
2. Garnish with olives and serve.

160 - Alkaline Veggie Juice

Servings: 2
Total Time: 5 minutes

Ingredients:
- 2 carrots
- 1 cucumber
- ¼ head green cabbage
- 1 cup kale
- ½ lemon
- ½ cup parsley
- 1 inch piece ginger
- 1 inch piece turmeric

Directions:
1. Place all ingredients in a juicer and serve immediately.

161 - Coconut Lime Smoothie

Servings: 1
Total Time: 5 minutes

Ingredients:
- 4 ounces fresh coconut meat
- ½ cup coconut water
- ½ cup coconut milk
- 1 tablespoon coconut oil
- 1 lime, peeled
- 1 banana, frozen
- 3 - 4 ice cubes
- ½ teaspoon lime zest

Directions:
1. Place all ingredients except the lime zest in a blender and blend on high until fully combined.
2. Garnish with lime zest and serve.

162 - Berry Blast Smoothie

Servings: 1
Total Time: 5 minutes

Ingredients:
- 1 cup spinach
- ¼ cup blueberries
- ¼ cup raspberries
- 1 tablespoon raw cashew butter
- 1 tablespoon ground flaxseed
- 1 tablespoon coconut oil
- 1 cup almond milk
- 1 tablespoon chia seeds
- 1 tablespoon hemp hearts

Directions:
1. Place all ingredients except the chia seeds and hemp hearts in a blender and combine.
2. Stir in chia and hemp hearts and serve.

163 - Minty Morning Shake

Servings: 2
Total Time: 5 minutes

Ingredients:
- ¾ cup unsweetened coconut milk
- ¼ cup canned coconut milk
- 1 cup fresh spinach
- ½ avocado
- ½ cup fresh mint leaves
- 2 bananas, frozen
- 2 dates, pitted
- 1 teaspoon vanilla extract
- ¼ teaspoon Himalayan salt
- ¼ teaspoon peppermint extract
- 6 - 8 ice cubes
- 1 teaspoon cacao nibs
- 2 fresh mint leaves

Directions:
1. Place all ingredients except the cacao nibs and 2 fresh mint leaves in a blender until smooth.
2. Garnish with cacao nibs and mint leaves before serving.

164 - Green Tea & Fruit Smoothie

Servings: 2
Total Time: 5 minutes

Ingredients:
- 2 ripe mangoes, peeled and chopped
- ½ cup raspberries
- ¼ cup pineapple, diced
- 1 ripe frozen banana, peeled
- 1 cup unsweetened almond milk
- 1 lime, juiced
- 2 teaspoons matcha green tea powder
- 3 - 4 ice cubes

Directions:
1. In a blender combine all ingredients until smooth and serve.

165 - Apple Pie Smoothie

Servings: 2
Total Time: 5 minutes

Ingredients:
- 1 red apple, cored and chopped
- ½ frozen banana
- 1 ½ cups unsweetened almond milk
- 3 dates, pitted, soaked for 15 minutes and drained
- 1 teaspoon cinnamon
- ½ teaspoon nutmeg
- ½ teaspoon vanilla extract
- ¼ teaspoon Himalayan salt

Directions:
1. In a blender combine all ingredients until smooth and serve.

166 - Morning Alkaline Lemon Water

Servings: 1
Total Time: 2 minutes

Ingredients:
- 8 ounces of alkaline water, either lukewarm or slightly warmed (not boiling)
- ½ lemon, juiced

Directions:
1. In a cup mix together the water and lemon juice.
2. Serve immediately either first thing upon waking (before consuming breakfast or other beverages) or before a meal.

167 - Detox Juice

Servings: 1
Total Time: 5 minutes

Ingredients:
- 2 small beets, peeled
- 1 carrot, peeled
- 1 small apple
- 1 lemon, peeled and seeds removed
- 1 ½ inch piece of ginger

Directions:
1. Place all ingredients in your juicer and serve immediately.

168 - Fruity Summer Lemonade

Servings: 2
Total Time: 2 minutes

Ingredients:
- 3 lemons
- 1 apple
- 1 ½ cups water
- 1 cup fresh strawberries, washed and hulled
- 1 cup watermelon, cubed
- ½ cup mint
- 1 teaspoon raw honey
- 5-6 ice cubes

Directions:
1. Juice lemons in a juicer and set aside the juice.
2. Juice apples in a juicer and combine juice with lemon juice in a blender.
3. Add water, strawberries, watermelon, mint, honey and ice cubes to the blender and blend until smooth.
4. Serve immediately.

169 - All Day Detox Water

Servings: 2
Total Time: 2 minutes

Ingredients:
- 16 ounces water
- 6 lemon slices
- 10 cucumber slices
- ¼ teaspoon Himalayan salt
- 5 - 6 ice cubes (optional)

Directions:
1. In a small pitcher, combine water, lemon, cucumber, salt and ice cubes (if using).

170 - Watermelon Mint Water

Servings: 2
Total Time: 2 minutes

Ingredients:
- 16 ounces water
- ½ cup watermelon, cubed
- 8 mint leaves, torn
- ¼ teaspoon Himalayan salt
- 5 - 6 ice cubes (optional)

Directions:
1. In a small bowl, using the back end of a spoon, muddle together the watermelon, mint and salt.
2. Add watermelon mint mixture to a pitcher and fill with water and ice cubes (if using).

171 - Glow Juice

Servings: 2
Total Time: 5 minutes

Ingredients:
- 2 green apples
- 1 cup collard greens, chopped
- 1 cup parsley
- ½ large cucumber
- 1 inch piece of ginger

Directions:
1. Place all ingredients in juicer. Serve juice immediately.

172 - Creamy Green Smoothie

Servings: 1
Total Time: 5 minutes

Ingredients:
- ½ cucumber
- 2 cups kale, stems removed
- ½ cup frozen broccoli
- ½ avocado
- 2 ounces silken tofu
- 1 inch ginger, grated
- 1 large lime, juiced
- ¼ teaspoon cayenne pepper
- ½ cup ice
- ½ cup unsweetened coconut milk

Directions:
1. Place all ingredients in blender and blend until smooth. Serve immediately.

173 - Creamy Orange Smoothie

Servings: 1
Total Time: 5 minutes

Ingredients:
- 3 medium oranges, peeled
- ½ banana, frozen
- ½ cup almond milk
- ½ teaspoon vanilla extract
- 1 ½ tablespoons raw honey
- 1 cup spinach
- ½ lime, juiced
- 2 cups ice cubes

Directions:
1. Place all ingredients in a high speed blender and combine. Serve immediately.

174 - Sunrise Juice

Servings: 1
Total Time: 5 minutes

Ingredients:
- 2 carrots, peeled
- 2 oranges, peeled
- 1 small beet, peeled
- 1 inch ginger

Directions:
1. In a juicer, juice together the carrots and oranges. Set aside.
2. Juice the beet and ginger in the juicer and place at the bottom of a glass. Slowly pour in the carrot and orange mixture. Serve immediately.

175 - Mulled Cider

Servings: 2
Total Time: 5 minutes

Ingredients:
- 1 apple seeded, cored and quartered
- 1 tablespoon raw honey
- ¼ orange peel with pith
- 1 inch piece ginger, grated
- ¼ teaspoon ground cinnamon
- Pinch of ground cloves
- Pinch of allspice
- Pinch of Himalayan salt
- 2 cups warm water

Directions:
1. Combine all ingredients in a high speed blender. Serve warm.

176 - Melon Melody

Servings: 2
Total Time: 5 minutes

Ingredients:
- 1 cup honeydew melon, cubed
- 1 cup watermelon, cubed
- 1 cup cantaloupe, cubed
- 3 - 4 mint leaves

Directions:
1. In a high speed blender, place all ingredients and combine until smooth.

177 - Mango Colada

Servings: 2
Total Time: 5 minutes

Ingredients:
- 1 cup frozen mango, cubed
- ½ banana, frozen
- 1 cup pineapple
- 1/2 cup unsweetened almond milk
- 1 can unsweetened coconut milk
- ½ lime, juiced
- 5 - 6 ice cubes

Directions:
1. In a high speed blender, place all ingredients and combine until smooth.

178 - Herbal Tonic

Servings: 2
Total Time: 10 minutes

Ingredients:
- 34 ounces water
- 1 lemon, peel grated and then juiced
- 2 teaspoons fresh thyme leaves
- 2 teaspoons fresh sage leaves
- 1 teaspoon rosemary leaves
- 2 inch piece ginger root, grated
- 1 inch piece turmeric root, grated
- 2 teaspoons apple cider vinegar
- 2 teaspoons raw honey

Directions:
1. In a small saucepan over medium heat, bring the water to a boil.
2. Add in lemon peel, lemon juice, thyme leaves, sage, rosemary, ginger, turmeric and vinegar. Simmer for 3 - 4 minutes.
3. Strain liquid into two mugs and stir a teaspoon of honey into each before serving.

179 - Probiotic Citrus Drink

Servings: 2
Total Time: 5 minutes

Ingredients:
- 2 large grapefruits, juiced
- 4 lemons, juiced
- 10 ounces water
- 1 teaspoon of acidophilus
- 1 clove of fresh garlic, grated
- 2 inches of fresh root ginger, grated
- 1 tablespoon olive oil
- 1 teaspoon matcha powder

Directions:
1. Add all ingredients to a blender and combine. Serve immediately.

180 - Acid Buster Juice

Servings: 2
Total Time: 5 minutes

Ingredients:
- 3 large kale leaves
- 2 celery stalks (and leaves)
- 1 cucumber
- 1 cup arugula
- ½ cup parsley
- ½ inch of fresh root ginger
- ½ lemon
- 8 ounces water
- 2 teaspoons apple cider vinegar

Directions:
1. Juice all ingredients in a juicer.

181 - Detox Stimulator Juice

Servings: 2
Total Time: 5 minutes

Ingredients:
- 1 cucumber
- 1 bunch kale
- 2 cups watercress
- 1 lemon
- 1 lime
- ½ grapefruit
- ½ inch ginger
- 1 small beetroot
- 1 small carrot

Directions:
1. Juice all ingredients in a juicer. Add up to ½ cup water if juice is too thick.

---

182 - Carrot Dream Smoothie

Servings: 1
Total Time: 5 minutes

Ingredients:
- 1 cup unsweetened almond milk
- 1 tablespoon almond butter
- ½ banana, frozen
- ½ inch fresh ginger, grated
- 1 teaspoon cinnamon
- ¼ teaspoon nutmeg
- 3 carrots, shredded
- 1 tablespoon chia seeds
- 1 teaspoon raisins

Directions:
1. Blend all ingredients except the chia seeds and raisins in a high speed blender until smooth and combined.
2. Stir in the chia seeds and garnish with raisins.

LUNCH RECIPES

183 - Southwest Stuffed Sweet Potatoes

Servings: 2
Total Time: 1 hour

Ingredients:
- 2 sweet potatoes
- 2 tablespoons of coconut oil
- ½ cup black beans, rinsed and drained
- 1 shallot, sliced
- 3 cups spinach
- Pinch of dried red chili flakes
- Pinch of cumin
- 1 avocado, peeled and sliced

Dressing
- 3 tablespoons olive oil
- 1 lime, juiced
- 1 teaspoon cumin
- Handful of cilantro, minced
- Salt and pepper

Directions:
1. Preheat oven to 400°F/205°C. Clean sweet potatoes and pierce several times with a fork. Place sweet potatoes on a baking tray lined with parchment paper and bake approximately 50 minutes or until soft.
2. Allow 5 minutes for sweet potatoes to cool.
3. While sweet potatoes are cooling heat skillet over medium heat and add coconut oil, shallot and black beans. Cook for 5 minutes then add spinach, dried chili flakes and cumin. Cook an additional 1 minute.
4. In a small bowl whisk together dressing ingredients.
5. Slice sweet potatoes down the middle and stuff with black bean mixture. Top with avocado slices.
6. Drizzle dressing over the sweet potatoes and serve.

184 - Coconut Cauliflower with Herbs & Spices

Servings: 2
Total Time: 30 minutes

Ingredients:
- ¼ cup coconut oil, melted
- ½ tablespoon ground cumin
- ¼ teaspoon ground coriander
- 1 teaspoon ground turmeric
- ¼ teaspoon black pepper, ground
- 1 large cauliflower, chopped into small florets
- 2 tablespoons pine nuts, toasted
- 1 tablespoon cilantro, minced
- ½ tablespoon mint, chopped roughly
- 1 tablespoon raisins
- Himalayan salt

Directions:
1. Preheat oven to 425°F/220°C. In a large bowl, mix together coconut oil, cumin, coriander, turmeric and black pepper. Fold in cauliflower and toss until well coated.
2. Spread cauliflower on baking tray and place in the oven for 20 minutes. Remove from oven and transfer to serving bowl.
3. Mix pine nuts, cilantro, mint, raisins and salt with the cauliflower and serve warm.

185 - Zoodles with Avocado Cream Sauce

Servings: 2
Total Time: 15 minutes

Ingredients:
- 1 tablespoon coconut oil
- 1 zucchini, spiralized
- 1 avocado, pitted and flesh removed
- 2 tablespoons olive oil
- ½ lemon, juiced
- 1 tablespoon water
- 2 tablespoons cilantro, minced and divided
- 1 teaspoon Himalayan salt
- ½ teaspoon black pepper, ground
- 2 tablespoons pepitas, toasted

Directions:
1. Melt coconut oil in a medium skillet over medium-high heat. Add zucchini noodles and cook 3-5 minutes. Turn off heat.
2. In a blender, combine the avocado, olive oil, lemon juice, water, 1 tablespoon cilantro, salt and pepper. Mix until well combined and creamy. If too thick, thin out with a little more water.
3. Add sauce to skillet with the zucchini noodles and toss to combine. If serving warm, turn heat to low and heat gently for 2 minutes.
4. Transfer to serving bowl and sprinkle with toasted pepitas and 1 tablespoon cilantro.

186 - Rainbow Pad Thai

Servings: 2
Total Time: 10 minutes

Ingredients:
- 3 medium zucchinis, spiralized
- 2 large carrots, shredded
- 3 scallions (green onions), sliced using green parts
- 1 cup red cabbage, shredded
- 1 cup broccoli, finely chopped
- 1 cup daikon radish (or other mostly white radish), shredded
- 1 cup of fresh cilantro, chopped
- 1 avocado, diced

Dressing
- 1 lime, juiced
- ¼ cup tahini
- 1 teaspoon sesame oil
- 1 garlic clove, minced
- 1 teaspoon ginger, minced

Directions:
1. Add first seven ingredients for salad into a large bowl and toss to combine.
2. Prepare dressing by whisking together all dressing ingredients until well combined and creamy.
3. Top vegetables with diced avocado and drizzle with dressing.

187 - Creamy Broccoli Slaw

Servings: 2
Total Time: 15 minutes

Ingredients:
- 1 head of broccoli
- ¼ cup raisins
- ¼ cup walnuts, chopped
- Pinch of salt
- Pinch of pepper

Dressing
- 3 tablespoons water
- 1 tablespoon tahini
- 2 teaspoons cumin
- 2 teaspoons coriander
- 1 teaspoon turmeric
- ½ teaspoon ground mustard
- ¼ teaspoon ginger
- 1 tablespoon coconut oil
- 1 tablespoon lemon juice

Directions:
1. Trim broccoli and chop into small florets. Set aside in a large bowl.
2. Prepare dressing by placing all dressing ingredients in a blender and blending until smooth and creamy.
3. Add raisins, walnuts, salt and pepper to broccoli and pour dressing over. Combine until all the broccoli mixture is evenly covered.

188 - Greek Vegetable Salad

Servings: 2
Total Time: 15 minutes

Ingredients:

- 2 red bell peppers, diced
- 3 large tomatoes, chopped
- 1 bunch kale (about 14 leaves), stems removed and sliced into thin ribbons
- 10 black olives in oil, sliced in half
- 1 red onion, halved and sliced
- 2 celery stalks, diced plus leaves
- 3 radishes, sliced
- ½ cup green or brown lentils, cooked

Dressing

- ½ cup lemon juice
- ¾ cup cold pressed olive oil
- 1 garlic clove, minced
- 1 teaspoon ground oregano
- 1 teaspoon dried basil
- ½ teaspoon ground cumin
- ¼ teaspoon sea salt
- ¼ teaspoon black pepper
- 1 teaspoon flaxseeds

Directions:

1. Combine the vegetables, olives & lentils in a bowl and set aside.
2. Place all dressing ingredients in a blender and blend until smooth and creamy.
3. Pour dressing over the vegetable mixture and lightly massage. Let rest at least 15 minutes before serving.

189 - Sweet & Spicy Vegetable Wrap

Servings: 2
Total Time: 30 minutes

Ingredients:

- 1 small red beet, peeled and diced small
- 1 small sweet potato, peeled and diced small
- 1 turnip, peeled and diced small
- 2 tablespoons olive oil
- 1 teaspoon Himalayan salt
- 1 teaspoon smoked paprika
- ¼ teaspoon cumin
- 2 sprouted grain tortilla wraps
- ½ cup arugula
- ½ cup sprouts

Dipping Sauce

- ½ cup unsweetened, plain yogurt
- 1 tablespoon lime juice
- 1 teaspoon cumin
- ½ teaspoon Himalayan salt
- ¼ teaspoon black pepper, crushed

Directions:

1. In a small bowl, combine dipping sauce ingredients and mix well. Set aside for at least 15 minutes.
2. On a baking tray lined with parchment paper place diced vegetables and drizzle with olive oil. Sprinkle with salt, paprika and cumin. Toss to combine and make sure vegetables are evenly coated. Place in oven at 375°F/190°C and roast 20 minutes.
3. Lay out each tortilla wrap and spread dipping sauce on top followed by the arugula and then the roasted vegetables.
4. Top with sprouts and roll up each wrap. Serve with extra dip on the side

190 - Mediterranean Millet Salad

Servings: 2
Total Time: 30 minutes

Ingredients:
- ½ cup millet, rinsed
- 1 cup water
- 12 cherry tomatoes, quartered
- 1 cucumber, diced small
- 1 scallion, sliced
- ½ cup black olives, quartered
- 1 cup parsley, chopped finely
- ¼ cup mint, chopped finely
- 2 tablespoons pine nuts, toasted

Dressing

- ¼ cup extra virgin olive oil
- 1 lemon, juiced
- 1 large garlic clove, minced
- 1 teaspoon dried oregano
- 1 teaspoon dried basil
- ½ teaspoon Himalayan salt

Directions:
1. Prepare millet by bringing water to a rolling boil in a saucepan over medium high heat. Stir in millet, reduce heat to low and put lid on the pan. Cook for approximately 20 minutes.
2. Whisk together dressing ingredients and set aside.
3. Combine millet, chopped vegetables, olives, parsley, mint and dressing in a large bowl. Gently toss to combine. Top with pine nuts and parsley for garnish.

---

191 - Grab & Go Zucchini Rolls

Servings: 2
Total Time: 20 minutes

Ingredients:
- 2 medium zucchinis, sliced very thin lengthwise using vegetable peeler
- 1 carrot, sliced into matchsticks
- 1 cucumber, sliced into matchsticks
- 2 radishes, sliced thinly
- ½ cup red cabbage, shredded
- 1 avocado, peeled and sliced
- 1 small bunch cilantro

Super Greens Hummus

- ½ cup chickpeas, drained and rinsed (or prepared fresh)
- ¼ cup soaked cashews
- 1 tablespoon tahini
- 1 cup kale leaves, de-stemmed and chopped
- ½ cup parsley
- 1 teaspoon of paprika
- 1 garlic clove
- ½ lemon, juiced
- 1/3 cup olive oil
- 1 teaspoon Himalayan salt

Directions:
1. Make the Super Greens Hummus by adding all the Super Greens Hummus ingredients to a blender or food processor and blending until creamy and smooth, adding more olive oil if the hummus is too thick.
2. Lay out each of the zucchini ribbons on a flat surface. Spread hummus on each of the zucchini ribbons. On top of the hummus add carrots, cucumber, radish, cabbage, avocado and some of the cilantro.
3. Begin rolling the one side of the zucchini ribbon until reaching the other end.

192 - Apple Kale Salad

Servings: 2
Total Time: 5 minutes

Ingredients:
- 3 cups kale, stems removed and sliced into thin ribbons
- 1 cucumber, diced
- 1 Granny Smith apple, cored and diced
- ½ cup cooked brown rice
- 1 avocado diced
- ¼ cup pomegranate seeds
- ½ cup walnuts, chopped

Dressing
- ¼ cup apple cider vinegar
- ¼ cup olive oil
- 3 tablespoons lemon juice
- 1 lemon, zested
- 1 teaspoon Himalayan salt
- ½ teaspoon black pepper, crushed

Directions:
1. Place kale, cucumber, apple, brown rice, avocado, pomegranate seeds and walnuts in a large bowl.
2. Whisk together dressing ingredients in a separate bowl until well combined.
3. Drizzle dressing over greens and toss to combine.

193 - Lentils & Greens Rice Pilaf

Servings: 2
Total Time: 10 minutes

Ingredients:
- ¼ cup vegetable broth
- ½ cup pak choi, sliced
- ½ cup broccoli florets
- 1 carrot, diced
- ½ lemon, juiced
- 1 cup of wild rice, cooked
- ½ cup green or brown lentils, cooked
- 1 cup arugula
- 1 teaspoon Himalayan salt
- 1 teaspoon black pepper, crushed
- 1 teaspoon crushed almonds
- 1 avocado

Directions:
1. Add vegetable broth to a medium skillet over medium high heat. Let it come to a slight simmer and add pak choi, broccoli, carrot and lemon juice. Cook for 5 minutes.
2. Turn heat off and stir in wild rice, lentils, arugula, salt, pepper and almonds.
3. Transfer to plates and top with avocado slices.

194 - Collard Wraps

Servings: 2
Total Time: 10 minutes

Ingredients:
- 2 large collard leaves
- ¼ cup brown rice, cooked
- ¼ cup purple cabbage, shredded
- ¼ cup carrots, shredded
- 1 zucchini, spiralized
- ¼ cup broccoli sprouts

Avocado Spread
- 1 avocado, mashed
- 1 tablespoon ground flaxseeds
- 1 tablespoon chia seed
- 1 teaspoon chili powder
- 1 garlic clove, minced
- ½ lemon, juiced
- 1 teaspoon Himalayan salt
- ½ teaspoon black pepper, crushed

Directions:
1. Make avocado spread by adding all the Avocado Spread ingredients to a bowl and combining well.
2. Open up the collard leaves on your work surface making sure each is flat and without many holes.
3. Spread avocado spread evenly over each wrap and top with brown rice. Add vegetables starting with the cabbage and ending with the sprouts.
4. Fold the bottom of the wrap and then fold in each side. Secure with a toothpick and enjoy.

195 - Sesame Greens & Tofu

Servings: 2
Total Time: 15 minutes

Ingredients:
- 1 ½ tablespoons toasted sesame oil
- 2 tablespoons olive oil
- 8 ounces extra firm tofu, cubed
- 2 cup broccoli florets, chopped finely
- ½ cup red bell pepper, diced
- 1 garlic clove, minced
- 2 tablespoons soy sauce or tamari
- ½ lemon, juiced
- 1 teaspoon sesame seeds

Directions:
1. Heat ½ tablespoon sesame oil and 1 tablespoon olive oil in a pan over medium low heat and add tofu. Cook for 10 minutes, turning occasionally. Set tofu aside and add 1 more tablespoon of olive oil and 1 tablespoon of sesame oil.
2. Stir in broccoli, red bell pepper and garlic. Cook for 5 minutes or until softened. Add tofu back to the pan and stir in soy sauce and lemon juice. Top with sesame seeds and serve.

196 - Roasted Carrot & Quinoa Salad

Servings: 2
Total Time: 25 minutes

Ingredients:
- 1 pound carrots, peeled and sliced into 1 inch pieces
- 1 teaspoon coconut oil, melted
- 1 teaspoon smoked paprika
- 1 teaspoon cumin
- 1 teaspoon chili powder
- ¼ teaspoon salt
- 2 cups arugula
- ½ cup quinoa, cooked
- 2 tablespoons pepitas, toasted
- 1 cup broccoli sprouts

Dressing
- 1 garlic clove, minced
- ¼ cup tahini
- 1 lemon, juiced
- 1 teaspoon turmeric
- ¼ teaspoon salt
- ¼ teaspoon black pepper, crushed
- 3 tablespoons water

Directions:
1. Preheat oven to 400°F/205°C. Toss carrots with coconut oil, paprika, cumin, chili powder and salt. Layer in an even layer on a baking tray lined with parchment paper. Bake for 20 minutes or until lightly browned, turning once.
2. While carrots are cooking, make dressing by combining all the dressing ingredients in a blender or food processor. Add more water if mixture is too thick.
3. In a large bowl, combine roasted carrots, quinoa, arugula and dressing together.
4. Top with pepitas and sprouts.

197 - Raw Fennel Salad with Citrus Dressing

Servings: 2
Total Time: 10 minutes

Ingredients:
- 1 pomegranate, seeds removed
- 1 cup carrots, grated
- 1 fennel bulb, halved and then sliced
- 1 grapefruit, segmented
- 1 tablespoon pumpkin seeds, toasted

Citrus Dressing
- 3 tablespoons fresh lime juice
- 5 tablespoons fresh orange juice
- 1 tablespoon olive oil
- 1 teaspoon apple cider vinegar
- ½ teaspoon nutmeg
- 1 teaspoon Himalayan salt
- 1 teaspoon black pepper, crushed

Directions:
1. In a large bowl, combine Citrus Dressing ingredients and whisk well.
2. Add to the large bowl the pomegranate seeds, carrots, fennel and grapefruit. Toss well to combine and garnish with pumpkin seeds.

198 - Taco Salad Bowl

Servings: 2
Total Time: 20 minutes

Ingredients:
- 2 cups kale, stems removed and sliced into thin ribbons
- 1 tablespoon olive oil
- 1 carrot, shredded
- 5 green onions, sliced
- 1 red bell pepper, sliced into strips
- 1 ½ cups cooked brown lentils
- ½ cup walnuts, toasted
- 1 tablespoon tomato paste
- 1 garlic clove, minced
- ½ teaspoon smoked paprika
- ½ teaspoon chili powder
- ½ teaspoon cumin
- ½ teaspoon Himalayan salt
- ¼ cup water
- ½ avocado, sliced

Cashew Ranch Dressing
- 1 ¼ cup cashews, soaked overnight and drained
- ½ cup water
- 1 lemon, juiced
- 1 teaspoon apple cider vinegar
- ¼ cup parsley
- 3 tablespoons chives, chopped
- 2 tablespoons fresh dill, chopped
- 1 teaspoon nutritional yeast
- 1 teaspoon Himalayan salt
- 1 teaspoon black pepper, crushed

Directions:
1. In a large bowl, place kale and drizzle with olive oil. Massage kale gently and set aside for 5 minutes before adding in the carrots, green onions and red bell pepper.
2. In a food processor add brown lentils, walnuts, tomato paste, garlic, smoked paprika, chili powder, cumin, salt and water to make taco "meat". Pulse together until crumbly.
3. Clean food processor and add ingredients for the Cashew Ranch Dressing. Process until smooth.
4. Place lentil & walnut "meat" on top of the vegetables, top with avocado slices and drizzle with Cashew Ranch dressing.

---

199 - Veggie & Mango Sushi

Servings: 2 (1 sushi roll per serving)
Total Time: 35 minutes

Ingredients:
- 2 nori sheets
- ½ zucchini, cut into thin strips
- 1 carrot, cut into thin strips
- 1 cup mango, cut into thin strips
- 1 cup sprouts
- 1 avocado, sliced

Cauliflower Rice
- ½ head cauliflower, cut into florets
- ½ tablespoon olive oil
- ½ cup quinoa, cooked and warmed
- ½ teaspoon tamari
- ½ teaspoon apple cider vinegar
- ½ teaspoon coconut aminos
- 1 teaspoon sesame seeds

Directions:
1. Process cauliflower florets in a food processor until a rice consistency is formed. Place cauliflower rice on a parchment paper lined baking tray, drizzle with olive oil and roast in an oven that has been preheated to 425°F/220°C for 25 minutes.
2. Place roasted cauliflower and warm quinoa in a large bowl and add tamari, vinegar, coconut aminos and sesame seeds. Combine well until it becomes sticky and holds together slightly when pushed together.
3. On a bamboo mat or tea towel in front of you, place a nori sheet and add half of the cauliflower rice at the end closest to you but leaving a slight space.
4. Place half of the zucchini, carrot, mango, sprouts and avocado on top of the rice. Roll up starting with the edge closest to you and pressing in as you go.
5. Repeat with the remaining nori, cauliflower rice and vegetables/fruit.
6. Slice each roll into 8 pieces and serve.

200 - Buddha Bowl

Servings: 2
Total Time: 35 minutes plus 5 hours in the fridge

Ingredients:
- 1 bunch kale, stems removed and sliced into thin ribbons
- 1 tablespoon olive oil
- 1 teaspoon lemon juice
- 2 cups quinoa, cooked
- 1 cup lentils, cooked
- 10 cherry tomatoes, halved
- 1 zucchini, made into noodles with a spiralizer
- 1 avocado, sliced
- 1 tablespoon black sesame seeds
- 1 tablespoon green onions, thinly sliced

Pickled Radishes
- 3 red radishes, thinly sliced
- ¼ cup apple cider vinegar
- ¼ cup water
- 1 tablespoon honey
- 1 teaspoon Himalayan salt
- ½ jalapeno, seeded and diced
- 1 teaspoon whole black peppercorns

Tahini Dressing
- ¼ cup tahini
- ¼ cup warm water
- 1 teaspoon lemon juice
- 1 tablespoon maple syrup
- ½ teaspoon turmeric
- 1 garlic clove, minced

Directions:
1. In a jar that has a lid, place in all Pickled Radishes ingredients. Mix well and let sit for 5 hours in the fridge with the lid on. Make sure the radishes are always covered with liquid.
2. Prepare Tahini Dressing by place all the ingredients in a small bowl and whisk together until smooth. If mixture is too thick, thin it out with more water.
3. Place kale in a large mixing bowl and massage gently with the olive oil and lemon juice. Let rest 10 minutes.
4. To assemble and serve, place kale at the bottom of a bowl and top with quinoa, lentils, tomatoes, zucchini noodles, avocado and pickled radishes. Drizzle with Tahini Dressing and sprinkle with black sesame seeds and green onions.

---

201 - Confetti Cauliflower Rice

Servings: 2
Total Time: 20 minutes

Ingredients:
- ½ cauliflower head, cut into florets
- 2 teaspoons olive oil
- 2 tablespoons red onion, chopped
- ¼ cup red bell pepper, chopped
- ¼ cup green bell pepper, chopped
- 1 garlic clove, minced
- 3 tablespoons water
- 1 teaspoon chili powder
- ¼ teaspoon ground cumin
- ½ teaspoon Himalayan salt
- ½ cup black beans
- ¼ cup cilantro, chopped
- 2 tablespoons green onions, thinly sliced

Directions:
1. Make cauliflower rice by processing the cauliflower florets in the food processor until it becomes a rice-like consistency.
2. Heat olive oil in a medium skillet over medium-low heat. Add onion, red bell pepper, green bell pepper and garlic. Cook for 5 minutes before adding the cauliflower rice, water, chili powder, cumin and salt.
3. Continue cooking another 5 minutes or until liquid is absorbed. Stir in black beans and cilantro and cook 2 minutes until warmed.
4. Garnish with green onions and serve.

202 - Creamy Sweet Salad

Servings: 2
Total Time: 20 minutes

Ingredients:
- ½ teaspoon coriander powder
- ¼ teaspoon cumin
- ¼ teaspoon turmeric
- ¼ teaspoon cinnamon
- ½ teaspoon Himalayan salt
- ½ teaspoon black pepper, crushed
- 1 cup unsweetened yogurt
- 2 tablespoons olive oil
- 2 cups steamed brown rice
- 3 cups celery, sliced into ½ inch pieces
- 1 cup red bell pepper, diced
- 1 cup pear, cored, peeled and cut into 1 inch pieces
- 2 tablespoons green onions, thinly sliced
- 2 tablespoons raisins
- 1 tablespoon almonds, slivered
- 4 cups mixed greens

Directions:
1. In a small bowl, combine the coriander, cumin, turmeric, cinnamon, salt and pepper. Add to the yogurt and olive oil to the spice mixture. Let sit for 15 minutes.
2. Place brown rice, celery, bell pepper, pear, green onions, raisins and almonds in a medium sized bowl. Pour yogurt mixture into the bowl and mix well to combine.
3. Serve brown rice and pear mixture over mixed greens.

203 - Sweet Spinach Salad

Servings: 2
Total Time: 15 minutes

Ingredients:
- ¾ cup carrots, shredded
- 1 tablespoon lime juice
- ½ cup unsweetened yogurt
- ½ cup apple, cored and diced into 1 inch pieces
- ¼ cup raisins
- ¼ cup walnuts, toasted and chopped
- 2 tablespoons parsley, chopped
- 4 cups spinach, chopped
- 1 teaspoon cinnamon
- 1 teaspoon nutmeg
- 1 teaspoon Himalayan salt
- 1 teaspoon black pepper, crushed

Directions:
1. Combine all ingredients in a large bowl and mix well.
2. Chill for 10 minutes before serving.

204 - Creamy Fruit Salad

Servings: 2
Total Time: 15 minutes

Ingredients:
- ¾ cup carrots, shredded
- 1 tablespoon lime juice
- ½ cup unsweetened yogurt
- ½ cup apple, cored and diced into 1 inch pieces
- ¼ cup raisins
- ¼ cup walnuts, toasted and chopped
- 2 tablespoons parsley, chopped
- 4 cups spinach, chopped
- 1 teaspoon cinnamon
- 1 teaspoon nutmeg
- 1 teaspoon Himalayan salt
- 1 teaspoon black pepper, crushed

Directions:
1. Combine all ingredients in a large bowl and mix well.
2. Chill for 10 minutes before serving.

205 - Steamed Green Bowl

Servings: 2
Total Time: 15 minutes

Ingredients:
- 1 tablespoon coconut oil
- 1 medium onion, finely sliced
- 1 garlic clove, minced
- 1 teaspoon turmeric
- 1 inch piece ginger, grated
- 1 head broccoli, cut into florets
- 1 large zucchini, sliced
- ½ cup green peas
- 2 cups coconut milk
- 1 cup cashews, ground
- 2 green onions, thinly sliced
- 1 teaspoon Himalayan salt
- 2 tablespoons cilantro, chopped

Directions:
1. Heat coconut oil in a medium saucepan over medium-low heat. Add onion, garlic, turmeric and ginger. Cook 5 minutes and then add broccoli, zucchini, peas and coconut milk.
2. Bring to a boil and then reduce heat to low and simmer for 15 minutes.
3. Stir in cashews, green onions, salt and cilantro and serve.

---

206 - Indian Cauliflower & Potato

Servings: 2
Total Time: 35 minutes

Ingredients:
- 2 tablespoons coconut oil
- 1 tablespoon ginger, grated
- 1 garlic clove, minced
- 1 medium onion, diced
- 3 tomatoes, diced
- ½ head of cauliflower, cut into florets
- ¼ cup green peas
- 5 yellow potatoes, diced
- 2 teaspoons turmeric
- 1 teaspoon cumin
- 1 teaspoon coriander
- 1 teaspoon ground cardamom
- ½ teaspoon cayenne pepper
- ½ teaspoon cinnamon
- 1 teaspoon Himalayan salt
- 1 teaspoon black pepper, crushed
- 3 cups water
- 2 tablespoons green onions

Directions:
1. Heat coconut oil in a medium saucepan over medium-low heat. Add ginger, onion, garlic and tomatoes. Cook for 5 minutes and then add cauliflower, peas, potatoes, turmeric, cumin, coriander, cardamom, cayenne, cinnamon, salt and pepper.
2. Continue cooking for 10 more minutes, stirring frequently. After 10 minutes, pour in water.
3. Cook mixture for 20 minutes or until vegetables are soft. Toss in green onions and serve.

---

207 - Berry & Vegetable Salad

Servings: 2
Total Time: 10 minutes

Ingredients:
- 2 tablespoons pumpkin seeds
- 1 tablespoon almonds, crushed
- 1 carrot, shredded
- ½ red bell pepper, sliced
- 1 tablespoon parsley, chopped
- 4 leaves of kale, stems removed and sliced into thin ribbons
- 1 shallot, sliced thinly
- 1 avocado
- 1 small cucumber, diced
- 3 tablespoons olive oil
- 1 lemon, juiced
- ½ head of red cabbage, shredded
- 1 cup alfalfa sprouts
- ½ small tangerine, sliced into segments
- ½ cup raspberries

Directions:
1. Add all ingredients to a large bowl. Toss well to combine and coat the vegetables with the oil and lemon juice.
2. Serve immediately.

208 - Shredded Cauliflower Salad

Servings: 2
Total Time: 10 minutes

Ingredients:
- ½ head of cauliflower, chopped into small pieces (like rice) in food processor
- 1 cup spinach, finely chopped
- 2-3 leaves kale, stems removed and finely chopped
- ¼ cup cilantro, finely chopped
- 2 green onions, sliced
- 1 tablespoon chives
- 1 ripe avocado, mashed
- 1 tablespoon tamari
- 1 teaspoon coconut aminos
- 1 lime, juiced
- ½ teaspoon red chili flakes
- 2 tablespoons cashews, toasted and crushed
- 2 tablespoons pumpkin seeds, toasted and crushed
- 1 tablespoon flaxseeds
- 1 teaspoon cayenne pepper
- 1 teaspoon cumin
- ½ teaspoon Himalayan salt
- 2 teaspoons coconut oil, melted
- 1 teaspoon raw honey

Directions:
1. In a large bowl, add cauliflower, spinach, kale, cilantro, green onions and chives.
2. Whisk together mashed avocado, tamari, coconut aminos, lime juice and chili flakes until smooth. Pour over the salad and massage gently.
3. In a small bowl, combine cashews, pumpkin seeds, flaxseeds, cayenne pepper, cumin, salt, coconut oil and honey together.
4. Top salad with the nut/seed mixture.

209 - Root Vegetable & Citrus Bowl

Servings: 2
Total Time: 50 minutes

Ingredients:
- ¼ cup orange juice
- ¼ cup grapefruit juice
- 1 teaspoon Dijon mustard
- 1 tablespoon apple cider vinegar
- 1 teaspoon coconut oil
- ½ teaspoon sea salt
- ½ teaspoon black pepper, crushed
- ¼ teaspoon cayenne pepper
- ½ red onion, quartered
- 1 sweet potato, cut into chunks
- 1 carrot, cut into chunks
- 1 small beet, peeled and cut into large chunks
- 2 garlic cloves, peeled and left whole
- ½ inch piece ginger, grated
- ¼ cup parsley, chopped
- 2 tablespoons rosemary
- 1 ½ cups quinoa, cooked
- 2 tablespoons parsley (for garnishing)
- 2 tablespoons pumpkin seeds

Directions:
1. Preheat oven to 400°F/205°C.
2. Whisk together the orange juice, grapefruit juice, mustard, vinegar, coconut oil, salt, pepper and cayenne in a small bowl.
3. In a large bowl combine the onion, potato, carrot, beet, garlic, ginger, parsley, rosemary. Pour citrus juice mixture over the vegetables and toss to coat.
4. Place vegetables on a parchment lined baking tray and place in the oven for 45 minutes, turning once.
5. Remove vegetables and place on top of quinoa. Garnish with parsley and pumpkin seeds and serve.

210 - Veggie Jambalaya

Servings: 2
Total Time: 5 minutes plus 6 hours slow cooker time

Ingredients:
- ½ eggplant, peeled and cut into ½ inch pieces
- 1 small zucchini, cut into ½ inch pieces
- 1 small yellow squash, cut into ½ inch pieces
- 1 celery stalk, diced
- ¼ cup olive oil
- ½ yellow onion, finely diced
- 1 garlic clove, minced
- 1 jalapeño, seeds removed and finely diced
- ½ red bell pepper, diced
- 2 small tomatoes, diced
- ⅛ teaspoon cayenne pepper
- ¼ teaspoon smoked paprika
- 1 teaspoon thyme
- 1 tablespoon apple cider vinegar
- 1 teaspoon Himalayan salt
- 1 teaspoon black pepper, crushed
- 2 cups water
- ½ uncooked brown rice
- 2 tablespoons green onions, sliced

Directions:
1. In a slow cooker, add all ingredients except the rice and green onions. Stir to combine and place lid on the slow cooker.
2. Cook on low for 5 hours.
3. After 5 hours, stir in the rice and ensure there is enough water to cover entire mixture. Cook another 40 minutes on low or until rice is tender.
4. Transfer to bowls and garnish with green onions.

211 - Detox Salad

Servings: 2
Total Time: 10 minutes

Ingredients:
- 3 beets, peeled, roasted and diced
- 3 green onions, sliced
- 1 lime, juiced
- ¼ cup raisins
- 3 cups watercress
- 1 pear, diced
- 1 celery stalk, diced
- ½ avocado, diced
- ½ cup almonds, toasted and crushed

<u>Dressing</u>
- 1 garlic clove, minced
- ¼ teaspoon Himalayan salt
- 1 teaspoon coriander
- 1 teaspoon cumin
- ½ teaspoon cinnamon
- ½ teaspoon turmeric
- ½ teaspoon fresh ginger, grated
- 1 lemon, juiced
- 6 tablespoons of avocado oil

Directions:
1. In a large bowl, combine beets, green onions, lime juice, raisins, watercress, pear, celery, avocado and almonds. Toss well to combine.
2. In a small bowl or jar, combine all the Dressing ingredients together. Whisk well to combine.
3. Pour Dressing over the beet and watercress mixture and toss well to coat.
4. Serve immediately.

212 - Alkaline Falafel Salad

Servings: 2
Total Time: 35 minutes

Ingredients:
- 2 cups kale, stems removed and thinly sliced
- 1 cup radicchio, sliced
- ½ cucumber, diced
- ½ tomato, diced
- 1 lemon, juiced
- 2 tablespoons olive oil
- 1 teaspoon Himalayan salt
- 1 teaspoon black pepper crushed
- ¼ cup pomegranate seeds
- 1 avocado, diced
- ¼ cup parsley, chopped

Falafels
- 1 teaspoon olive oil
- ½ red onion, diced
- 1 garlic clove, minced
- ½ cup brown lentils, cooked
- ¼ cup chickpeas
- ¼ cup peas, cooked
- ¼ cup parsley, chopped
- ¼ cup tablespoons tahini
- ¼ teaspoon cumin
- 1 teaspoon Himalayan salt

Directions:
1. Preheat oven to 375°F/190°C.
2. Make the Falafels by heating a teaspoon of olive oil in a medium skillet over medium heat. Add the onion and garlic and cook 5 minutes until soft. Add to a food processor along with the lentils, chickpeas, peas and parsley. Pulse until mixture starts to come together, then add the tahini, cumin and salt.
3. Form Falafels by forming into balls using 1 ½ tablespoons of the mixture and placing on a baking tray lined with parchment paper. Bake the Falafels for 15-20 minutes.
4. In a large bowl, combine the kale, radicchio, cucumber, tomato, lemon juice, olive oil, salt and pepper. Toss to coat well.
5. Place Falafels, pomegranate seeds, avocado and parsley on top of the salad and serve immediately.

213 - Chopped Salad

Servings: 2
Total Time: 10 minutes

Ingredients:
- ½ head romaine lettuce
- 1 cucumber, diced
- 1 tomato, diced
- ½ green bell pepper, diced
- ¼ cup green onions, diced
- ¼ cup black olives, chopped
- 2 tablespoons red onion, diced
- 2 tablespoons parsley, chopped

Dressing
- 1 tablespoon lemon juice
- 2 tablespoons apple cider vinegar
- 1 garlic clove, minced
- ¼ teaspoon Himalayan salt
- ⅛ teaspoon pepper
- ½ teaspoon dried oregano
- 1/3 cup olive oil

Directions:
1. Make Dressing by whisking together all the Dressing ingredients together.
2. Place the lettuce, cucumber, tomato, bell pepper, green onions, olives, red onion and parsley in a large bowl. Drizzle with Dressing and toss to coat.

214 - Carrot & Quinoa Bowl

Servings: 2
Total Time: 30 minutes

Ingredients:
- 1 cup warm water
- 1 tablespoon miso
- 1 tablespoon olive oil
- 1 bunch carrots, scrubbed and cut into large chunks
- 1 fennel bulb, thinly sliced
- 2 cups quinoa, cooked
- ½ lemon, juiced
- 3 tablespoons parsley, chopped
- ¼ teaspoon Himalayan salt
- 2 tablespoons black sesame seeds
- 2 tablespoons green onions, sliced

Directions:
1. Whisk together water and miso in a small bowl
2. Heat olive oil in a large skillet over medium heat. Add carrots and fennel bulb in a single layer and cook 3 minutes before flipping. Continue to cook for another 3 minutes.
3. Pour miso and water mixture into the pan and reduce heat to low. Cook, with the lid on, for 20 minutes.
4. While carrots are cooking, combine the quinoa, lemon juice, parsley and salt in a medium bowl.
5. Place cooked carrot and fennel mixture over the quinoa, sprinkle with the sesame seeds, green onions and serve.

---

215 - Seaweed & Carrot Rollups

Servings: 2
Total Time: 35 minutes

Ingredients:
- ¼ ounce dried wakame
- 1 carrot, spiralized
- 8 ounces extra-firm tofu, drained and cut into 2 long rectangles
- ½ avocado, pitted, peeled and thinly sliced
- 2 sprouted tortillas or large lettuce leaves (such as Bibb lettuce)
- 1 tablespoon sesame seeds
- 1 tablespoon green onion, sliced

Dressing
- 1 teaspoon reduced-sodium tamari
- 1 teaspoon coconut aminos
- 1 teaspoon toasted sesame oil
- ¼ teaspoon red chili flakes

Directions:
1. In a large bowl, place wakame and cover with cold water. Let sit for 10 minutes and then drain and dry.
2. In a small bowl, stir together the tamari, coconut aminos, sesame oil and red chili flakes to form the Dressing.
3. Place half the wakame, carrot, tofu and avocado in one of the wraps or lettuce leaves. Drizzle the Dressing on top and sprinkle with sesame seeds and green onion.
4. Repeat with the remaining ingredients and roll up each one. Secure with a toothpick and serve.

216 - Middle Eastern Salad

Servings: 2
Total Time: 15 minutes

Ingredients:
- 4 small eggplants, sliced into ⅛ inch thick rounds
- 1 teaspoon Himalayan salt
- 1 tablespoon olive oil
- ½ cup lentils, cooked
- ½ cup parsley, chopped
- ½ cup dill, chopped
- ¼ cup walnuts, toasted
- ¼ cup raisins
- 1 ½ cups arugula
- 1 ½ cups spinach
- 1 lemon, zested and juiced
- 3 tablespoons olive oil
- ½ teaspoon Himalayan salt
- ½ teaspoon black pepper, crushed

Spice Blend

- ¼ cup sesame seeds, toasted
- 2 tablespoons dried thyme
- 1 tablespoon dried marjoram
- 1 tablespoon dried oregano
- ½ teaspoon Himalayan salt

Directions:
1. Place eggplant rounds on a paper towel and sprinkle with the teaspoon of salt. Allow to rest while continuing with the other directions.
2. While eggplant rests, prepare Spice Blend by combining all the Spice Blend ingredients in a small bowl and mixing well.
3. Brush eggplant with olive oil on both sides and sprinkle with Spice Blend. Place in a grill pan that has been preheated over medium-high heat. Cook for 5 minutes on each side or until tender.
4. In a small bowl, combine the lentils, parsley, dill, walnuts and raisins. Place on top of the arugula and spinach that has been combined in a large serving bowl. Squeeze lemon juice and drizzle olive oil on top and season with salt and pepper. Toss well to combine.
5. Place eggplant slices on top of the greens and lentil mixture and serve.

217 - Tropical Tofu Salad

Servings: 2
Total Time: 10 minutes

Ingredients:
- ½ mango, diced
- ½ cup pineapple, diced
- 1 carrot, shredded
- ½ red bell pepper, thinly sliced
- 7 ounces firm tofu, drained and diced
- ¼ cup cilantro, chopped
- 1 cup arugula
- ¼ cup sesame seeds, toasted
- 2 tablespoons green onions

Dressing

- 1 tablespoon white miso paste
- 2 teaspoons warm water
- 2 teaspoons coconut aminos
- 1 lime, juiced
- ¼ teaspoon cayenne pepper

Directions:
1. Make Dressing by combining the Dressing ingredients in a small bowl and whisking well. If mixture is too thick or miso won't dissolve, add more warm water.
2. In a large bowl, combine the mango, pineapple, carrot, bell pepper, tofu, cilantro and arugula together.
3. Drizzle Dressing on top and toss to coat.
4. Sprinkle with sesame seeds and green onions.

218 - Sweet Broccoli Quinoa Bowl

Servings: 2
Total Time: 10 minutes

Ingredients:
- 5 tablespoons water
- 2 tablespoons tahini
- 1 teaspoon turmeric
- ½ teaspoon cinnamon
- ½ lemon, juiced
- 1 teaspoon maple syrup
- 1 head broccoli, florets finely chopped
- ¼ cup red grapes, halved
- ¼ cup almonds, chopped
- 1 cup quinoa, cooked
- 1 teaspoon Himalayan salt
- 1 teaspoon black pepper, crushed

Directions:
1. In a small bowl, whisk together the water, tahini, turmeric, cinnamon, lemon juice and maple syrup until smooth.
2. In a large bowl, combine the broccoli, grapes, almonds and quinoa.
3. Pour tahini sauce over the broccoli and quinoa mixture and add salt and pepper.
4. Toss well to coat and serve.

219 - Cooling Mint Salad

Servings: 2
Total Time: 10 minutes

Ingredients:
- 2 cups spinach, chopped
- 2 cups radishes, thinly sliced
- 1 cucumber, diced
- 2 small red onions, cut in half and thinly sliced
- ¼ cup almonds, sliced

Mint & Citrus Dressing
- 1 tablespoon raw honey
- ¼ cup orange juice
- 1 tablespoon lemon juice
- 4 tablespoons olive oil
- 1 teaspoon Himalayan salt
- 1 teaspoon black pepper, crushed
- 1 cup fresh mint leaves, chopped

Directions:
1. In a small bowl, whisk together the Mint & Citrus Dressing ingredients.
2. In a large bowl, combine the spinach, radishes, cucumber, red onion and almonds. Pour in Mint & Citrus Dressing and toss to coat.
3. Serve immediately.

220 - Antioxidant Salad

Servings: 2
Total Time: 10 minutes

Ingredients:
- 1 tablespoon coconut oil
- 1 teaspoon apple cider vinegar
- ¾ cup almonds, toasted
- 1 garlic clove, minced
- ½ cup quinoa, cooked
- 1/3 cup raisins
- ¼ cup blueberries
- 2 cups spinach, torn
- 1 handful of sesame seeds
- 1 teaspoon Himalayan salt

Directions:
1. In a large bowl, toss together all ingredients and mix well.
2. Chill 5 minutes and serve.

221 - Minted Quinoa Salad

Servings: 2
Total Time: 5 minutes

Ingredients:
- ½ cup red quinoa, cooked
- ½ red bell pepper, diced
- ½ green bell pepper, diced
- ½ cucumber, diced
- 6 ounces chickpeas, cooked
- 1/3 cup mint leaves, thinly sliced
- ½ red onion, thinly sliced
- 2 tablespoons parsley, chopped
- 1 tablespoon pine nuts, toasted

Dressing
- 3 tablespoons olive oil
- 2 tablespoons lemon juice
- 1 tablespoon lemon zest
- ½ teaspoon Himalayan salt
- 1 teaspoon oregano

Directions:
1. In a large bowl, combine quinoa, red and green bell peppers, cucumber, chickpeas, mint leaves and onion.
2. In a small bowl, whisk together the olive oil, lemon juice, lemon zest, salt and oregano.
3. Pour Dressing over the quinoa and vegetables.
4. Garnish with parsley and pine nuts before serving.

222 - Sweet & Sour Seaweed Salad

Servings: 2
Total Time: 10 minutes plus 20 minutes soaking time

Ingredients:
- 3 tablespoons arame, soaked 10 minutes and then drained
- 1 tablespoon wakame, soaked 10 minutes and then drained
- 3 beets, grated
- 1 white radish, grated
- 1 shallot, sliced
- 2 cups spinach, chopped
- ½ cup mango, diced
- 2 tablespoons dried cherries, soaked 20 minutes and drained
- 2 tablespoons black sesame seeds
- ½ avocado, sliced

Dressing
- ½ cup white miso
- ¼ cup apple cider vinegar
- 1 lemon, juiced
- 3 tablespoons ginger, minced
- 1 garlic clove, minced
- ¼ cup avocado oil
- 1 tablespoon maple syrup
- Few drops of toasted sesame oil

Directions:
1. In a large bowl, combine arame, wakame, beets, radish, shallot, spinach, mango and cherries.
2. In a blender, combine the Dressing ingredients until well combined.
3. Pour Dressing over the seaweed mixture, garnish with the sesame seeds and avocado and serve immediately.

223 - Nutty Snap Pea & Quinoa Salad

Servings: 2
Total Time: 10 minutes

Ingredients:
- 1 tablespoon extra-virgin olive oil
- 1 lemon, zested and juiced
- 1 tablespoon orange juice
- ⅛ teaspoon red chili flakes
- ⅛ teaspoon salt
- ⅛ teaspoon black pepper, crushed
- 1 ½ cup snap peas
- 1 cup quinoa, cooked
- ½ red onion, thinly sliced
- ¼ cup mint leaves, thinly sliced
- 1 tablespoon almonds, slivered and toasted
- 1 tablespoon pine nuts, toasted

Directions:
1. In a small bowl, whisk together the olive oil, lemon juice and zest, orange juice, red chili flakes, salt and black pepper.
2. Combine the snap peas, quinoa, red onion and mint. Pour olive oil and citrus juice mixture over the quinoa and snap peas and toss to combine.
3. Garnish with almonds and pine nuts before serving.

---

224 - Grab & Go Green Wraps

Servings: 2
Total Time: 10 minutes

Ingredients:
- 1 cup green peas, steamed
- 1 small avocado
- 1 small lime, juiced
- ¼ cup fresh cilantro leaves, chopped
- 1 shallot, diced
- ¼ - ½ jalapeño pepper, seeds removed and diced
- ¼ teaspoon Himalayan salt
- 4 large collard greens
- ½ red bell pepper, seeds removed and thinly sliced
- 1 carrot, julienned

Directions:
1. In a food processor or blender, combine the peas, avocado, lime, cilantro, shallot, jalapeno and salt. Process until combined but still has some texture.
2. Lay out a collard green in front of you and spread pea avocado mixture on top. Add some bell pepper and carrot strips. Roll up the collard green and secure with a toothpick.
3. Repeat with remaining ingredients and serve.

---

225 - Autumn Salad

Servings: 2
Total Time: 35 minutes

Ingredients:
- 1 large sweet potato, diced
- 2 beets, peeled and diced
- 2 tablespoons coconut oil
- ¼ teaspoon Himalayan salt
- 1 teaspoon black pepper
- ¼ cup almonds, toasted and chopped
- ¼ cup raisins
- 1 cup spinach, chopped
- ½ cup quinoa, cooked
- ¼ cup parsley, chopped

Dressing
- 2 tablespoons raw apple cider vinegar
- 1 lime, juiced
- ¼ cup extra virgin olive oil
- 1 teaspoon Himalayan salt

Directions:
1. Preheat oven to 350°F/180°C.
2. In a small bowl, whisk together the vinegar, lime juice, olive oil and salt. Set aside.
3. Place diced sweet potato and beets in a small bowl and pour in the coconut oil and sprinkle with salt and pepper. Toss well to coat and then arrange on a baking tray that has been lined with parchment paper.
4. Roast the potato and beet in the oven for 25 minutes or until tender.
5. In a large bowl, combine the sweet potato, beet, almonds, raisins, spinach, quinoa and parsley. Pour Dressing on top and toss well to coat.
6. Serve immediately.

226 - Nutty Tacos

Servings: 2
Total Time: 10 minutes

Ingredients:
- ½ cup walnuts
- ¼ cup slivered raw almonds, blanched
- ¼ cup sun-dried tomatoes, soaked, drained, and roughly chopped
- 2 tablespoons olive oil
- 1 teaspoon ground cumin
- 1 teaspoon ground coriander
- ⅛ teaspoon chili powder
- ⅛ teaspoon garlic powder
- ⅛ teaspoon onion powder
- ⅛ teaspoon smoked paprika
- 1 teaspoon coconut aminos
- 1 teaspoon tamari
- ⅛ teaspoon Himalayan salt
- ¼ cup red quinoa, cooked
- 4-6 romaine lettuce leaves
- 2 tablespoons nutritional yeast
- 1 tablespoon chopped flat-leaf cilantro

Directions:
1. Place walnuts and almonds in a food processor and pulse until chopped. Add in the sun-dried tomatoes and pulse a few times until mixed with the walnuts and almonds and mixture is crumbly.
2. Add in the olive oil, cumin, coriander, chili, garlic, onion, paprika, coconut aminos, tamari and salt. Pulse a few more times until combined.
3. Place nut and tomato mixture in a bowl and stir in the quinoa.
4. Divide mixture up amongst the romaine leaves and top with nutritional yeast and cilantro before serving.

227 - Cold Sesame Salad

Servings: 2
Total Time: 15 minutes

Ingredients:
- 1 tablespoon avocado oil
- 1 large sweet potato, spiralized into noodles
- 1 large zucchini, spiralized into noodles
- 3 tablespoons tahini paste
- 1 ½ tablespoons toasted sesame oil
- 2 tablespoons raw apple cider vinegar
- 1 teaspoon raw honey
- 1 teaspoon lime juice
- 1 teaspoon coconut aminos
- 1 teaspoon tamari
- Pinch crushed red pepper flakes
- ⅛ teaspoon Himalayan salt
- 1 green onion, diced
- 1 tablespoon sesame seeds

Directions:
1. Heat avocado oil in a medium skillet over medium heat. Add sweet potato noodles and cooked 5 minutes, stirring occasionally. Add zucchini noodles and cook another 3 minutes before turning the heat to low.
2. Whisk together the tahini, sesame oil, apple cider vinegar, honey, lime juice, coconut aminos, tamari and red pepper flakes in a small bowl.
3. Pour tahini mixture over the noodles and toss to coat. Season with the salt and transfer to serving bowl.
4. Let chill and then garnish with green onions and sesame seeds to serve.

228 - Tex-Mex Bowl

Servings: 2
Total Time: 20 minutes plus 5 hours chill time

Ingredients:
- 4 bell peppers, seeds and stems removed, sliced into strips
- 1 large red onion, thinly sliced
- 2 large garlic cloves, minced
- 2 oranges, juiced
- 1 lemon, zested and juiced
- 1 lime, zested and juiced
- ¼ cup apple cider vinegar
- ¼ cup olive oil
- ¼ teaspoon Himalayan salt
- 1 avocado, sliced
- 2 tablespoons cilantro
- 2 tablespoons nutritional yeast

- 1 teaspoon Himalayan salt
- 1 teaspoon paprika
- ½ teaspoon cayenne pepper
- ½ teaspoon garlic powder
- ½ cup black beans, drained and rinsed

Salsa

- 2 large tomatoes, diced
- ½ red onion, peeled and diced
- ¼ cup cilantro leaves, diced
- ¼ teaspoon salt
- juice of 1 lime

Spiced Brown Rice

- 1 cup brown rice, cooked
- 2 teaspoons chili powder
- 1 ½ teaspoon garlic powder

Directions:
1. In a large bowl, combine the bell peppers, red onion, garlic, orange juice, lemon juice and zest, lime juice and zest, vinegar, olive oil and salt. Cover and let rest in the fridge for 5 hours.
2. While peppers marinate in the fridge, make the Salsa by combining all the Salsa ingredients in a small bowl. Stir well to combine, cover and place in the fridge.
3. In a medium sized bowl, add together all the Spiced Brown Rice ingredients. Toss well and set aside.
4. Heat a medium sized skillet over medium-high heat. Add bell peppers and a few tablespoons of the marinade. Sauté for 10 minutes or until the bell peppers and onions are soft.
5. Place rice in serving bowls and top with bell pepper/onion mixture, sliced avocado, salsa and garnish with cilantro and nutritional yeast.

---

229 - Stuffed Eggplant

Servings: 2
Total Time: 25 minutes

Ingredients:
- 2 small eggplants, cut into ½ inch thin slices
- 2 tablespoons olive oil, divided
- 1 shallot, diced
- 1 teaspoon cumin
- ¼ teaspoon turmeric powder
- ¼ teaspoon cinnamon
- 1 tablespoon fresh ginger, grated

- ⅛ teaspoon cayenne pepper
- 1 large carrot, diced
- 1 cup quinoa, cooked
- 2 tablespoons raisins
- 1 tablespoon pine nuts, toasted
- 3 tablespoons parsley, chopped

Directions:
1. Prepare eggplant by brushing with 1 tablespoon of the olive oil and placing on a grill pan or a baking tray. Broil in the oven on high for 4 minutes each side. Remove and set aside.
2. In a medium skillet over medium-low heat, add the shallot and cook for 3 minutes.
3. Add the cumin, turmeric, cinnamon, ginger and cayenne. Sauté for 1 minute before adding in the carrot. Continue cooking for another 8 minutes.
4. Transfer shallot and carrot mixture to a medium sized bowl and add the quinoa, raisins, pine nuts and parsley.
5. Place a small amount of the quinoa filling on each eggplant slice and roll up, securing with a toothpick before serving.

230 - Chickpea Millet & Cucumber Salad

Servings: 2
Total Time: 10 minutes

Ingredients:
- 1 garlic clove, minced
- 1 teaspoon cumin
- 1 teaspoon Himalayan salt
- 3 tablespoons avocado oil
- 2 tablespoons lemon juice
- 1 teaspoon lemon zest
- 1 teaspoon oregano
- 1 cup millet, cooked
- 1 cup cucumber, diced
- 1 cup chickpeas, drained + rinsed
- 3 cups spinach, chopped
- 2 tablespoons parsley, chopped
- 2 tablespoons black olives, chopped

Directions:
1. In a small bowl, whisk together the garlic, cumin, salt, avocado oil, lemon juice, lemon zest and oregano to create the dressing. Set aside.
2. Combine the millet, cucumber, chickpeas, spinach and parsley in a large bowl. Pour dressing over the millet mixture and toss well to coat.
3. Garnish with black olives

231 - Sweet Brussel Sprout Salad

Servings: 2
Total Time: 55 minutes

Ingredients:
- ½ pound brussel sprouts, washed, trimmed, and halved
- 1 shallot, diced
- 1 teaspoon Himalayan salt
- ½ cup vegetable broth
- 2 tablespoons olive oil
- 1 lemon, zested
- 1 pear, cored and diced
- 1 cup almonds, toasted and chopped
- 1 teaspoon dried thyme
- ¼ teaspoon cinnamon
- 1 cup quinoa, cooked

Directions:
1. Preheat the oven to 350°F/180°C.
2. Place brussel sprouts in a deep baking dish and add in shallot and salt. Pour in vegetable broth and drizzle with olive oil.
3. Bake the brussel sprouts for 30 minutes before adding in the lemon zest, pear, almonds, thyme and cinnamon. Toss well to combine and bake for another 15 minutes.
4. In a large bowl, combine the quinoa and brussel sprout mixture and serve immediately.

232 - Cherry & Fennel Salad

Servings: 2
Total Time: 10 minutes

Ingredients:
- 1 cup quinoa, cooked
- 1 cup dark red cherries, pitted and halved
- 1 cup spinach, chopped
- ½ bulb fennel, thinly sliced
- ¼ cup almonds, toasted and crushed
- 1 teaspoon Himalayan salt
- 1 teaspoon black pepper, crushed
- 2 tablespoons olive oil
- 2 tablespoons apple cider vinegar
- 1 garlic clove, minced

Directions:
1. In a large bowl, combine the quinoa, cherries, spinach, fennel and almonds.
2. Whisk together the salt, pepper, olive oil, vinegar and garlic in a small bowl.
3. Pour olive oil mixture over the quinoa and toss to coat. Serve immediately.

233 - Brussel Sprouts Bowl

Servings: 2
Total Time: 35 minutes

Ingredients:

- 1 bunch brussel sprouts, halved
- 1 small red onion, sliced thinly into half-moon shapes
- 2 tablespoons ghee, melted
- 1 cup brown rice, cooked
- ½ cup walnuts, chopped
- 2 tablespoons raisins
- 2 tablespoons pomegranate seeds
- 1 teaspoon Himalayan salt
- 1 teaspoon black pepper
- 1 tablespoon parsley, chopped

Directions:

1. Preheat oven to 400°F/205°C. On a baking tray, place brussel sprouts and red onion. Drizzle with ghee and roast in the oven for 30 minutes or until brussel sprouts are crispy.
2. Place brussel sprouts, brown rice, walnuts, raisins and pomegranate seeds in a large bowl. Season with salt and pepper.
3. Garnish with parsley and serve warm.

234 - Spicy Mexican Salad

Servings: 2
Total Time: 15 minutes

Ingredients:

- 1 teaspoon coconut oil
- 1 red onion, chopped
- 1 green bell pepper, diced
- 2 garlic cloves, minced
- 1 cup quinoa, cooked
- ¼ teaspoon cayenne pepper
- ¼ teaspoon chili powder
- ⅛ teaspoon red chili flakes
- 1 teaspoon cumin
- 1 teaspoon Himalayan salt
- 1 teaspoon black pepper, crushed
- 1 15 ounce cans black beans, rinsed and drained
- 2 teaspoons lime juice
- ½ cup chopped fresh cilantro
- 1 avocado, sliced

Directions:

1. In a medium skillet over medium heat, add the oil, red onion and green bell pepper. Cook 5 minutes or until the onion and pepper are soft. Add the garlic and cook another 2 minutes.
2. Place quinoa, cayenne pepper, chili powder, chili flakes, cumin, salt and pepper in the pan and stir well. Cook 3 minutes before adding the black beans.
3. Continue to cook black bean and quinoa mixture for 5 minutes. Turn the heat off and stir in the lime juice and cilantro.
4. Transfer to serving bowls and garnish with avocado slices.

235 - Chilled Avocado Soup with Salmon

Servings: 2
Total Time: 10 minutes

Ingredients:

- 3 ripe avocados, pitted and flesh removed
- 1 small shallot, chopped
- 1 tablespoon green onion, sliced
- 4 tablespoons lemon juice, divided
- 2 tablespoons full fat coconut cream
- 1 ½ cups vegetable broth
- ¼ teaspoon cumin
- ¼ teaspoon Himalayan salt
- 1 can salmon, drained and flaked
- 1 teaspoon olive oil
- 1 teaspoon black pepper, crushed
- 2 tablespoons cilantro, divided

Directions:

1. In a blender combine the avocado, shallot, green onion, 2 tablespoons of lemon juice, coconut cream, vegetable broth, cumin and salt. Let chill for at least 1 hour.
2. In a small bowl, combine the salmon, olive oil, black pepper, 2 tablespoons lemon juice and 1 tablespoon cilantro.
3. Place chilled avocado soup in bowls and top each with salmon, remaining cilantro. Serve immediately.

236 - Asian Pumpkin Salad

Servings: 2
Total Time: 40 minutes

Ingredients:
- 1 tablespoon white sesame seeds
- 1 tablespoon black sesame seeds
- ¼ teaspoon ground cloves
- ¼ teaspoon ground garlic
- ¼ teaspoon ground mustard
- ¼ teaspoon red chili flakes
- ½ teaspoon Himalayan salt, divided
- 2 cups pumpkin, cubed
- 1 ½ tablespoons olive oil
- 4 cups kale, stems removed and sliced into thin ribbons
- 1 tablespoon lemon juice
- ¼ cup pomegranate seeds
- ½ avocado, diced

Directions:
1. Preheat oven to 400°F/205°C. Line a baking tray with parchment paper.
2. On a large plate, combine the white and black sesame seeds, cloves, garlic, mustard, chili flakes and half the salt.
3. Drizzle pumpkin with 1 tablespoon olive oil and then roll each cube into the sesame seed mixture, pressing slightly to coat. Place pumpkin cubes on the parchment paper and bake for 30 minutes, turning once.
4. While pumpkin cooks, add kale to a large bowl and drizzle with remaining olive oil, lemon juice and remaining salt. Massage gently for 3 minutes and set aside.
5. When pumpkin is done, place on top of the kale and garnish with pomegranate seeds and avocado.

237 - Squash & Sprouts Salad

Servings: 2
Total Time: 55 minutes

Ingredients:
- 1 small butternut squash, cubed
- 2 small apples, cored and chopped
- 2 shallots, sliced
- 1 cup brussel sprouts, halved
- 2 tablespoons avocado oil
- ¼ teaspoon cinnamon
- ⅛ teaspoon turmeric
- 1 teaspoon Himalayan salt
- 1 teaspoon black pepper, crushed
- 1 tablespoon walnuts, toasted and chopped
- 1 tablespoon parsley, chopped

Directions:
1. Preheat oven to 400°F/205°C. Line a baking tray with parchment paper.
2. In a large bowl, combine the butternut squash, apples, shallots, brussel sprouts, avocado oil, cinnamon, turmeric, salt and pepper. Spread on baking tray in a single layer.
3. Roast in the oven for 45 minutes or until vegetables are tender, tossing halfway through.
4. Remove from oven and transfer to serving platter.
5. Sprinkle with walnuts and parsley before serving.

238 - Fennel Citrus Salad

Servings: 2
Total Time: 10 minutes

Ingredients:
- 1 small orange, segmented
- ½ small red grapefruit, segmented
- 2 small fennel bulbs, thinly sliced
- 1 tablespoon mint, chopped
- ½ cup parsley, chopped
- 2 tablespoons fresh lemon juice
- 2 tablespoons fresh orange juice
- ¼ cup olive oil
- ⅛ teaspoon sea salt
- ½ teaspoon freshly ground black pepper
- 2 tablespoons pomegranate seeds
- ½ avocado, diced

Directions:
1. In a large bowl, combine the orange segments, grapefruit segments, fennel slices, mint and parsley.
2. Whisk together lemon juice, orange juice, olive oil, salt and pepper. Pour over the citrus and fennel mixture. Toss well to coat.
3. Transfer to plate and garnish with pomegranate seeds and avocado. Serve immediately.

239 - Mushroom Wraps

Servings: 2
Total Time: 10 minutes

Ingredients:
- 1 cup shiitake mushrooms, sliced
- 1 cup cremini mushrooms, sliced
- ½ cup zucchini, shredded
- ¼ cup coconut aminos
- 2 tablespoons tamari
- 3 garlic cloves, minced
- 1 tablespoon sesame oil
- ¼ teaspoon red chili flakes
- 4 Boston lettuce leaves
- 1 carrot, shredded
- 1 tablespoon cilantro
- 1 tablespoon cashews, crushed

Sauce
- ¼ cup raw coconut aminos
- 1 tablespoon raw honey
- ¼ teaspoon hot chili oil
- 1 teaspoon sesame oil
- 1 teaspoon red chili flakes
- ¼ teaspoon Himalayan salt

Directions:
1. In a large bowl, combine both mushrooms, zucchini, coconut aminos, tamari, garlic, sesame oil and chili flakes. Let sit while you prepare the Sauce.
2. To prepare the Sauce, whisk together the Sauce ingredients in a small bowl.
3. Assemble wraps by placing some of the mushroom mixture in a lettuce leaf and top with some carrot, cilantro and cashews. Drizzle sauce on top. Repeat with remaining ingredients and serve.

---

240 - Sweet Potato Wraps

Servings: 2
Total Time: 25 minutes

Ingredients:
- 4 collard greens
- ½ cup quinoa, cooked
- 1 cup spinach
- ½ red onion, thinly sliced
- 1 cup alfalfa sprouts
- 1 avocado

Sweet Potato Hummus
- 1 large sweet potato, peeled and cubed
- 1/3 cup of tahini
- ¼ cup of olive oil
- ½ lemon, juiced
- 1 garlic clove, minced
- ¼ teaspoon chili powder
- ⅛ teaspoon cinnamon powder
- ¼ teaspoon Himalayan salt
- ¼ teaspoon black pepper, crushed

Directions:
1. Place sweet potatoes in a medium saucepan and cover with water. Bring to a boil over medium-high heat and then reduce heat to a simmer and cook 15 minutes or until potatoes are tender.
2. Drain water from the sweet potatoes and place sweet potatoes in a food processor along with the tahini, olive oil, lemon juice, garlic, chili powder, cinnamon, salt and pepper. Process until smooth.
3. Lay out each of the collard greens before you and spread each with the Sweet Potato Hummus. Top with quinoa, spinach, onion, sprouts and avocado. Roll up and secure with toothpicks if necessary. Repeat with remaining collard greens and filling.

241 - Refresh Green Grape Salad

Servings: 2
Total Time: 5 minutes

Ingredients:
- 1 cup arugula
- 1 cup watercress
- 1 beet, shredded
- 1 cup red cabbage, shredded or chopped
- ½ avocado, diced
- 10 green grapes, halved or whole
- ½ cup walnuts, crushed
- 2 tablespoons olive oil
- ½ lemon, juiced
- ½ teaspoon Himalayan salt
- ½ teaspoon black pepper, crushed

Directions:
1. Place the arugula, watercress, beet, cabbage, avocado, grapes and walnuts in a large bowl.
2. Drizzle with olive oil, lemon juice, salt and pepper. Toss well to coat and serve immediately.

242 - Fall Lentil Salad

Servings: 2
Total Time: 25 minutes

Ingredients:
- 1 small delicata squash, sliced into ½ inch thick slices
- 2 tablespoons olive oil
- 2 teaspoons thyme leaves, chopped
- 1 garlic clove, minced
- 1 tablespoon apple cider vinegar
- 1 tablespoon lemon juice
- ½ tablespoon maple syrup
- ½ teaspoon Himalayan salt
- ½ teaspoon black pepper, crushed
- ½ cup lentils, cooked
- 2 cups spinach, stems removed and thinly sliced
- 2 tablespoons pine nuts, toasted

Directions:
1. Preheat oven to 400°F/205°C. Line a baking tray with parchment paper. In a small bowl, combine the squash, 1 tablespoon olive oil, thyme and garlic. Move the squash to the baking tray and bake in the oven for 20 minutes, flipping once halfway through.
2. Whisk together the remaining tablespoon olive oil, apple cider vinegar, lemon juice, maple syrup, salt and pepper.
3. In a large bowl combine the lentils, spinach, baked squash and pine nuts. Drizzle with olive oil mixture, toss to coat and serve immediately.

243 - Brown Rice & Sprouts Salad

Servings: 2
Total Time: 5 minutes

Ingredients:
- 1 cup brown rice, cooked
- 1 ½ cups of quinoa, cooked
- ½ yellow bell pepper, diced
- 5 cherry tomatoes, halved
- 2 tablespoons cilantro, chopped
- 2 tablespoons parsley, chopped
- 1 cup alfalfa sprouts
- 2 tablespoons almonds, toasted
- 1 tablespoon raisins

Dressing
- 3 tablespoons olive oil
- 1 tablespoon apple cider vinegar
- 1 tablespoon lemon juice
- 1 teaspoon maple syrup
- 1 garlic clove, minced

Directions:
1. In a large serving bowl, place brown rice and top with quinoa, yellow pepper, tomatoes, cilantro, parsley, sprouts, almonds and raisins.
2. Whisk together Dressing ingredients in a small bowl and pour over the salad.
3. Toss before serving.

244 - Chopped Beet & Quinoa Salad

Servings: 2
Total Time: 40 minutes

Ingredients:
- 2 medium beets, ends cut and halved
- 1 cup quinoa, cooked
- 1 stalk celery, diced small
- ½ head red cabbage, shredded
- 1 garlic clove, minced
- 1 tablespoon apple cider vinegar
- 2 tablespoons olive oil
- ½ teaspoon Himalayan salt
- ¼ teaspoon black pepper, crushed
- ¼ cup fresh mint, chopped
- ¼ cup parsley, chopped

Directions:
1. Fill a medium saucepan (fitted with a steamer basket) with water until it reaches halfway. Bring water to a boil over medium heat and then add beets to the steamer basket. Cover with a lid and reduce heat to low and cook for 30 minutes or until beets are tender.
2. Remove beet skins by placing in a towel and rubbing off the skins. Chop the cooked beets into a small dice.
3. In a large bowl, combine quinoa, beets, celery, cabbage, garlic, vinegar, olive oil, salt, pepper, mint and parsley. Combine well and serve immediately.

245 - Sweet Quinoa Salad

Servings: 2
Total Time: 5 minutes

Ingredients:
- 3 cups spinach, chopped
- 1 cup quinoa, cooked
- 1 shallot, thinly sliced
- 2 apples, diced
- 2 tablespoons raisins
- 2 tablespoons walnuts, toasted and crushed
- 1 handful sprouts
- 2 tablespoons avocado oil
- ½ lemon, juiced
- ½ teaspoon Himalayan salt
- ⅛ teaspoon cinnamon
- ¼ teaspoon black pepper, ground

Directions:
1. Combine spinach, quinoa, shallot, apples, raisins, walnuts and sprouts in a large bowl.
2. Drizzle with avocado oil and pour in lemon juice. Add salt, cinnamon and black pepper.
3. Toss well to combine and serve immediately.

246 - Warm Spinach Salad

Servings: 2
Total Time: 15 minutes

Ingredients:
- 1 tablespoon coconut oil
- ½ cup red onion, sliced thinly
- 1 garlic clove, minced
- 5 cherry tomatoes, halved
- 6 cups baby spinach
- ½ teaspoon grated lemon peel
- ½ teaspoon Himalayan salt
- ½ teaspoon black pepper
- ¼ teaspoon cinnamon
- 1 cup brown rice, cooked
- 1 tablespoon pine nuts, toasted

Directions:
1. In a medium skillet over medium heat, melt coconut oil and add onion. Cook 5 minutes and then add the garlic, cooking for an additional 1 minute.
2. Add in tomatoes and spinach. Season with lemon peel, salt, pepper and cinnamon. Cook for 5 minutes or until spinach is wilted.
3. Place brown rice in a bowl and top with the spinach and tomato mixture.
4. Garnish with pine nuts and serve.

247 - Veggie Ramen

Servings: 1
Total Time: 15 minutes

Ingredients:
- 1 tablespoon of miso paste
- 1 inch ginger piece, minced
- 1 tablespoon tamari
- ½ lime, juiced
- ½ bell pepper, thinly sliced
- ¼ head of broccoli, cut into small florets
- 1 carrot, spiralized into noodles
- 4 mushrooms, stems removed and sliced
- ½ cup spinach
- ½ zucchini, spiralized
- 3 cups boiling water
- 1 tablespoon cilantro

Directions:
1. In a large bowl that has a lid, add the miso, ginger, tamari, lime juice, bell pepper, broccoli, carrot, mushrooms, spinach and zucchini.
2. Pour boiling water into the pot, stir well a few times and then place the lid on top.
3. Let sit 5 minutes and then garnish with cilantro and serve.

248 - Spicy Ginger Salad

Servings: 2
Total Time: 10 minutes

Ingredients:
- 3 cups kale
- 1 cup tomatoes, finely diced
- 1 tablespoon parsley, finely chopped
- 1 tablespoon raw sesame seeds
- 1 tablespoon raw pumpkin seeds
- 1 tablespoon almonds
- 1 garlic clove, minced
- ¼ teaspoon lemon zest
- ¼ teaspoon ginger, grated
- ⅛ teaspoon red chili flakes

Dressing
- 3 tablespoons olive oil
- 1 tablespoon lemon juice
- 1 tablespoon apple cider vinegar
- ¼ teaspoon fresh ginger juice
- ½ teaspoon Himalayan salt
- ¼ teaspoon cayenne pepper
- ¼ teaspoon black pepper, crushed

Directions:
1. Make the Dressing by combining the Dressing ingredients in a small bowl until well combined.
2. In a large bowl, combine the kale, tomatoes, parsley, sesame seeds, pumpkin seeds, almonds, garlic, lemon zest, ginger and chili flakes.
3. Pour Dressing over the kale and tomato mixture. Let rest 5 minutes before serving.

249 - Curry Squash Soup

Servings: 2
Total Time: 25 minutes

Ingredients:
- 1 tablespoon olive oil
- 1 shallot, sliced
- 1 yellow squash, diced
- ½ cup broccoli, cut into florets
- 1 teaspoon ginger, grated
- ½ teaspoon Himalayan salt
- ½ teaspoon black pepper, crushed
- ½ teaspoon cumin
- ½ teaspoon coriander
- ½ teaspoon cardamom
- ½ teaspoon turmeric
- ¼ teaspoon cinnamon
- 1 ½ cups vegetable broth
- ½ cup water
- 1 lemon, juiced
- 1 tablespoon cilantro, chopped
- 1 teaspoon pepitas, toasted

Directions:
1. Heat oil in a medium-sized pot over medium heat. Add shallot, squash, broccoli, ginger, salt, pepper, cumin, coriander, cardamom, turmeric and cinnamon.
2. Sauté 10 minutes until vegetables are softened and then add the broth, water and lemon juice. Let come to a low boil and then reduce heat to low and simmer 10 minutes.
3. Let cool 5 minutes and then transfer to a food processor or blender and blend until smooth.
4. Top with cilantro and pepitas to serve.

---

250 - Sweet Potato Nacho Boat

Servings: 2
Total Time: 35 minutes

Ingredients:
- 2 sweet potatoes
- ½ tablespoon balsamic vinegar
- ½ teaspoon coconut aminos
- ½ tablespoon apple cider vinegar
- ½ teaspoon cayenne pepper
- ¾ cup tempeh, diced
- 1 cup spinach
- 4 black olives, sliced
- 1 tomato, diced
- 1 shallot, diced
- ½ avocado, diced

Cheese Sauce

- ¼ head of cauliflower, steamed
- ½ cup nutritional yeast
- ½ cup vegetable broth
- 1 garlic clove, minced
- ¼ teaspoon cayenne pepper
- 1 tablespoon white miso
- 1 tablespoon lemon juice
- 1 teaspoon tahini
- ½ teaspoon chili powder

Directions:
1. Preheat oven to 400°F/205°C. Line a baking tray with parchment paper. Pierce sweet potatoes with a fork a few times and place on tray. Bake in the oven for 30 minutes.
2. Prepare Cheese Sauce by placing Cheese Sauce ingredients in a food processor or blender and mixing until smooth. Set aside.
3. In a small skillet over medium heat, add balsamic vinegar, coconut aminos, apple cider vinegar and cayenne. Let heat for 3 minutes and then add tempeh, tossing to coat. Cook 5 minutes until tempeh is warm and sauce is slightly reduced.
4. Cut open each sweet potato and add spinach, tempeh, olives, tomato, shallot and avocado. Drizzle cheese sauce on top and serve immediately.

251 - Spicy Orange Sweet Potato Bowl

Servings: 1
Total Time: 40 minutes

Ingredients:
- 1 medium sweet potato, cubed
- 2 teaspoons sesame seed oil
- 1 date, pitted and soaked 10 minutes and drained
- 3 tablespoon orange juice
- 1 tablespoon tamari
- 1 tablespoon coconut aminos
- 1 garlic clove, grated
- ½ teaspoon red chili flakes
- ½ teaspoon ginger, grated
- 2 cups broccoli, cut into florets, steamed
- 1 tablespoon sesame seeds

Directions:
1. Preheat oven to 400°F/205°C and place sweet potato on a baking tray lined with parchment paper. Coat sweet potato with 1 teaspoon sesame seed oil and then bake in the oven for 30 minutes.
2. In a blender, combine the date, orange juice, tamari, coconut aminos, garlic, red chili flakes and ginger. Set aside.
3. In a medium skillet, heat remaining sesame oil over medium-low and add steamed broccoli. Cook 3 minutes and set aside.
4. Add orange juice mixture to the pan and let come to a low simmer. Add the sweet potato and toss to coat. Cook 5 minutes until sauce is reduced slightly.
5. Serve sweet potato alongside the broccoli and garnish with sesame seeds.

252 - Cauliflower Colcannon

Servings: 2
Total Time: 5 minutes

Ingredients:
- 1 cauliflower, cut into florets and steamed
- ½ cup parsley, chopped
- 1 garlic clove, chopped
- 1 tablespoon lemon juice
- 2 tablespoon olive oil
- ½ teaspoon Himalayan salt
- 1 cup brussel sprouts, shredded
- 1 cup green cabbage, thinly shredded
- 1 tablespoon green onions, sliced

Directions:
1. Place steamed cauliflower, parsley, garlic clove, lemon juice, olive oil and salt in a food processor and blend until smooth.
2. Add the brussel sprouts and cabbage to the food processor and pulse 3-4 times so that the sprouts and cabbage are incorporated but not completely pureed.
3. Transfer to a bowl and garnish with green onion.

253 - Peas & Rice

Servings: 2
Total Time: 10 minutes

Ingredients:
- 3 tablespoons coconut oil
- 2 red chilies, chopped
- 2 garlic cloves, chopped
- ½ teaspoon fresh ginger, grated
- 1 shallot, sliced
- 1 pound green beans
- 3 tablespoons coconut milk
- 1 tablespoon unsweetened, shredded coconut
- ½ teaspoon Himalayan salt
- ½ teaspoon cayenne pepper
- 1 cup brown rice, cooked

Directions:
1. In a medium sized skillet over medium heat add coconut oil, chilies, garlic, ginger and shallots. Cook for 5 minutes and then add green beans, coconut milk, shredded coconut, salt and pepper.
2. Reduce heat to low and cook 5 minutes.
3. Serve on top of brown rice.

254 - Sweet & Spicy Sweet Potato Skillet

Servings: 2
Total Time: 25 minutes

Ingredients:
- 1 tablespoon olive oil
- ½ red onion, sliced
- 2 sweet potatoes, cubed
- ½ teaspoon cayenne pepper
- ½ teaspoon red chili flakes
- ½ teaspoon cumin
- ½ teaspoon Himalayan salt
- ½ teaspoon black pepper, crushed
- 1 apple, cored and cubed
- 1 cup chickpeas, cooked
- ½ cup quinoa, cooked
- ¼ cup walnuts, toasted and crushed
- 1 teaspoon raw honey
- 2 tablespoons cilantro, chopped

Directions:
1. Heat oil in a medium skillet over medium-high heat and add onions. Cook 5 minutes and then add sweet potato, cayenne, chili flakes, cumin, salt and pepper.
2. Cook for 15 minutes until tender and crispy, stirring frequently.
3. Add in apple and cook 2 minutes and then add chickpeas, quinoa, walnuts and honey.
4. Garnish with cilantro and serve warm.

255 - Broccoli & Pear Salad

Servings: 2
Total Time: 20 minutes

Ingredients:
- 1 head of broccoli, shredded into very small florets
- 1 pear, cored and chopped
- ¼ red onion, thinly sliced
- 2 tablespoons cup walnuts, crushed
- 2 tablespoons cup pepitas
- ¼ cup raisins

Dressing

- ¾ cup unsweetened yogurt
- 2 tablespoons apple cider vinegar
- 1 tablespoon lemon juice
- 1 tablespoon honey
- ¼ teaspoon Himalayan salt

Directions:
1. In a large bowl, combine the broccoli, pear, red onion, walnuts, pepitas and raisins.
2. Whisk together the Dressing ingredients in a small bowl and pour over broccoli mixture.
3. Toss well to coat and let sit in the fridge for 10 minutes before serving.

256 - Quinoa Nicoise Salad

Servings: 1
Total Time: 10 minutes

Ingredients:
- 2 cups kale, stems removed and thinly sliced
- 1 teaspoon lemon juice
- ½ cup quinoa, cooked
- 1 cup green beans, cut in half and steamed
- ¼ cup black olives, sliced
- ½ cup sweet potato, diced and steamed
- 1 small tomato, diced
- 1 tablespoon olive oil
- ¼ teaspoon Himalayan salt
- ¼ teaspoon black pepper, crushed

Directions:
1. Place kale in a large bowl and add lemon juice. Gently massage the kale and then let sit for 5 minutes.
2. After 5 minutes, place kale on a large plate and top with quinoa, green beans, olives, sweet potato and tomato.
3. Drizzle with olive oil and season with salt and pepper.

257 - Red & Green Salad

Servings: 1
Total Time: 10 minutes

Ingredients:
- 1 cup quinoa, cooked
- 2 cups fresh baby spinach, chopped
- 2 cups arugula
- 1 pint strawberries, hulled and sliced
- 1 avocado, diced
- ¼ cup pepitas, toasted
- 1 shallot, thinly sliced

Dressing
- 1/2 cup avocado oil
- 3 tablespoons apple cider vinegar
- 1 tablespoon honey
- ½ teaspoon Himalayan salt
- ½ teaspoon black pepper, crushed

Directions:
1. In a small bowl, whisk together the Dressing ingredients and set aside.
2. Combine quinoa, spinach, arugula, strawberries, avocado, pepitas and shallot in a large bowl.
3. Pour dressing over and toss well to coat.

258 - Shredded Kale Salad

Servings: 2
Total Time: 5 minutes

Ingredients:
- 1 cup brussel sprouts, finely shredded
- 1 cup kale, stems removed and finely chopped
- 1 cup red cabbage, finely shredded
- ¼ cup wild rice, cooked
- ¼ cup almonds
- ¼ cup pomegranate seeds
- 1 tablespoon olive oil
- 1 lime, juiced
- 2 teaspoons apple cider vinegar
- 1 teaspoon honey
- ½ teaspoon Himalayan salt
- ¼ teaspoon black pepper

Directions:
1. Combine all ingredients in a large bowl and toss to coat well.
2. Serve immediately.

259 - Italian Kale Stew

Servings: 2
Total Time: 30 minutes

Ingredients:
- 1 tablespoon olive oil
- ½ medium onion, finely diced
- 2 garlic cloves, chopped
- 1 teaspoon dried oregano
- ½ teaspoon dried thyme
- 1 ½ cups chickpeas, cooked
- 1 tomato, diced
- 1 tablespoon tomato paste
- 3 cups vegetable broth
- 3 cups kale, stems removed and finely chopped
- ¼ cup fresh parsley, chopped
- ½ teaspoon Himalayan salt

Directions:
1. Heat oil in a large pot over medium heat. Add onion, garlic, oregano and thyme. Cook 7 minutes.
2. Add chickpeas, tomato, tomato paste and vegetable broth. Bring to a boil and then reduce heat to a simmer and cook for 20 minutes.
3. Stir in kale and let it wilt before stirring in parsley and salt.
4. Serve immediately.

260 - Spinach & Beet Salad

Servings: 2
Total Time: 5 minutes

Ingredients:
- 4 cups spinach, chopped
- ½ cup fresh parsley, chopped
- 1 cup quinoa, cooked
- 1 cup beets, cooked and grated
- 1 cup lentils, cooked

Dressing
- 1 lemon, juiced
- 2 tablespoons tahini
- 1 tablespoon warm water
- ½ teaspoon Himalayan salt
- ½ teaspoon black pepper

Directions:
1. In a small bowl, whisk together the Dressing ingredients.
2. Place spinach, parsley, quinoa, beets and lentils in a large bowl and pour in the Dressing.
3. Toss well to coat and serve immediately.

261 - Spicy Cabbage Bowl

Servings: 2
Total Time: 10 minutes

Ingredients:
- 2 teaspoons sesame oil
- ½ teaspoon fresh ginger, grated
- 1 teaspoon garlic, minced
- 1 cup brown rice, cooked
- 1 cup cabbage kimchi, chopped
- 2 teaspoons tamari
- 1 teaspoon coconut aminos
- 2 cups kale, stems removed and finely chopped
- ¼ cup green onion
- 1 tablespoon sesame seeds

Directions:
1. Heat sesame oil in a medium skillet over medium heat and add ginger, garlic, brown rice, kimchi, tamari and coconut aminos.
2. Let cook 5 minutes and then add in the kale and green onions. Toss well to combine and cook 4 minutes.
3. Garnish with sesame seeds before serving.

262 - Fennel Citrus Salad

Servings: 2
Total Time: 10 minutes

Ingredients:
- 1 small orange, segmented
- ½ small red grapefruit, segmented
- 2 small fennel bulbs, thinly sliced
- ½ cup parsley, chopped
- 1 tablespoon mint, chopped
- 2 tablespoons fresh lemon juice
- 2 tablespoons fresh orange juice
- ¼ cup olive oil
- ⅛ teaspoon sea salt
- ½ teaspoon freshly ground black pepper
- 2 tablespoons pomegranate seeds
- ½ avocado, diced

Directions:
1. In a large bowl, combine the orange segments, grapefruit segments, fennel slices, mint and parsley.
2. Whisk together lemon juice, orange juice, olive oil, salt and pepper. Pour over the citrus and fennel mixture. Toss well to coat.
3. Transfer to plate and garnish with pomegranate seeds and avocado. Serve immediately.

DINNER RECIPES

263 - Salmon & Vegetable Kebabs with Greens Pesto

Servings: 2
Total Time: 30 minutes

Ingredients:
- 6 ounces wild, fresh salmon, skin removed and cut into 1 inch cubes
- 1 small zucchini, chopped into 1 inch pieces
- 12 cherry tomatoes
- 1 small yellow pepper, cut into 1 inch pieces
- ½ sweet onion, quartered and divided into 12 pieces
- 1 tablespoon olive oil
- 1 garlic clove, minced
- ½ teaspoon Himalayan salt
- ¼ teaspoon black pepper, crushed
- 4 wooden skewers, soaked in water for at least 30 minutes

Pesto Sauce
- 1 cup spinach
- 1 garlic clove, minced
- ½ cup basil leaves
- ¼ cup pumpkin seeds
- ¼ cup olive oil
- 1 teaspoon Himalayan salt
- ½ teaspoon pepper
- 1 lemon, juiced

Directions:
1. Thread salmon and vegetables on skewers in desired pattern. Place skewers on a baking tray. Brush kebabs with olive oil, garlic, salt and pepper.
2. Place skewers in an oven that has been preheated to 400°F/205°C and bake for approximately 20 minutes, turning once and making sure fish is cooked through.
3. In a blender or food processor, place the ingredients for the Pesto Sauce and combine until smooth, adding more olive oil if too thick. Drizzle over cooked skewers.

264 - Coconut Curry & Vegetables

Servings: 2
Total Time: 25 minutes

Ingredients:
- 2 tablespoons coconut oil
- ½ yellow onion, diced
- 1 teaspoon fresh ginger, grated
- 2 medium zucchinis, cubed into 1 inch pieces
- 1 yellow bell pepper, cut into 1 inch pieces
- ½ cup eggplant, cubed into 1 inch pieces
- ¼ pound green beans, cut into 1 inch pieces
- 8 ounces firm tofu, cut into 1 inch pieces
- 1 tomato, diced
- 1 cup coconut milk
- 1/3 cup water
- 1 teaspoon Himalayan salt
- 2 teaspoons curry powder
- 3 tablespoons cilantro, chopped

Directions:
1. In a medium skillet heat coconut oil and add onion, ginger, zucchini, bell pepper, eggplant and beans. Cook for 5 minutes before adding the tofu and tomatoes. Let sauté for another 5 minutes.
2. Add coconut milk, water, salt, and curry powder. Let simmer 10 minutes. Stir in cilantro before serving.

265 - Loaded Spaghetti Squash

Servings: 2
Total Time: 40 minutes

Ingredients:
- 1 spaghetti squash, cut in half lengthwise and seeds removed
- 1 ½ tablespoons olive oil
- 1 leek, chopped
- 1 garlic clove, minced
- 6 tomatoes, diced
- 1 cup cooked green or brown lentils
- ½ teaspoon oregano
- ½ teaspoon Himalayan salt
- 1 cup basil leaves, torn
- ½ teaspoon lemon zest

Directions:
1. Rub 1 tablespoon of the olive oil on each of the spaghetti squash halves and place face down on a baking tray lined with parchment paper. Place in a 375°F/190°C oven for 30 minutes or until squash are tender.
2. In a skillet, heat remaining ½ tablespoon olive oil and add the leek, garlic and tomatoes. Cook 8 minutes before adding in the lentils and dried oregano. Continue to cook for another 5 minutes before seasoning with salt.
3. Remove squash from oven and with a fork using lengthwise strokes, separate the flesh. Add in the vegetable and lentil mixture and combine. Top with torn basil leaves, drizzle with any olive oil and lemon zest.

266 - Asian Noodle Bowl

Servings: 2
Total Time: 15 minutes

Ingredients:
- 4 ounces buckwheat soba noodles
- ½ cup broccoli florets, finely chopped
- ¼ head red cabbage, cored and thinly sliced
- ½ cup brussel sprouts, cored and thinly sliced
- 1 large carrot, shredded
- 1 scallion, sliced
- 2 tablespoons sesame seeds, toasted
- 1 tablespoon cilantro, chopped

Dressing

- ½ tablespoon ginger, minced
- 1 garlic clove, minced
- ½ tablespoon toasted sesame oil
- 2 teaspoons olive oil
- 2 tablespoons tamari
- 2 tablespoons coconut aminos
- ½ lime, juiced
- pinch of red pepper flakes

Directions:
1. Cook soba noodles according to package directions. Strain and rinse with cold water. Set aside.
2. Make the Dressing by combining all Dressing ingredients and whisking well. Place vegetables and soba noodles in a large bowl and mix well to combine.
3. Pour dressing over the noodles and vegetables. Sprinkle with sesame seeds, cilantro and serve.

267 - Spicy Marinara Sauce & Pasta

Servings: 2
Total Time: 25 minutes

Ingredients:
- 8 ounces spelt pasta
- 3 tablespoons olive oil
- 1 garlic clove, minced
- 1 shallot, diced
- 1 celery stalk plus greens, diced
- 1 carrot, diced
- 2 cups cherry tomatoes, diced
- ½ cup sun dried tomatoes, diced
- ½ small zucchini, diced
- ½ cup black olives, sliced
- 1 chili pepper, seeded and diced
- 1 teaspoon Himalayan salt
- 1 teaspoon black pepper, crushed
- 1 cup basil leaves, torn

Directions:
1. Cook spelt noodles according to package directions. Drain and set aside.
2. Add oil to a medium skillet over medium heat and sauté the garlic and shallot for 3 minutes before adding the celery and carrot. Cook for an additional 8 minutes, stirring occasionally. Toss in cherry tomatoes, sun dried tomatoes and zucchini. Cook another 3 minutes. Stir in olives, chili pepper, salt and pepper.
3. Toss pasta into the saucepan making sure to combine it thoroughly. Transfer to serving plate and top with basil leaves.

268 - Lemon Baked Fish Over Green Salad

Servings: 2
Total Time: 30 minutes

Ingredients:
- 8 ounces of wild salmon, cut into 2 fillets (skin on)
- ½ cup parsley, chopped
- ½ cup fresh basil, chopped
- 1 lemon, juiced
- 1 garlic clove, chopped
- 1 teaspoon cayenne pepper
- 1 tablespoon nutritional yeast
- 2 tablespoons olive oil
- 1 teaspoon sea salt
- 1 teaspoon black pepper, crushed
- ¼ cup pine nuts
- 4 lemon slices

Salad
- 3 cups kale, stems removed and sliced into thin ribbons
- 3 tablespoons olive oil
- 1 lemon, juiced
- 1 teaspoon Himalayan salt
- 1 cucumber, diced
- ¼ cup pepita seeds, toasted
- ½ avocado, diced

Directions:
1. Combine all ingredients except for the salmon and 4 lemon slices in a blender or food processor to form the greens mixture (add more olive oil if it is too thick).
2. Place salmon on a parchment lined baking tray. Top each fillet with greens mixture and place 2 lemon slices on each piece. Bake salmon in a preheated 375°F/190°C oven for approximately 15-20 minutes or until fish flakes easily and is cooked all the way through.
3. Place kale in a bowl and top with olive oil, lemon juice and salt. Massage the kale leaves until tender and set aside for 5 minutes before adding cucumber, pepitas and avocado.
4. Serve fish alongside salad.

269 - Cauliflower & Tahini Bowl

Servings: 2
Total Time: 30 minutes

Ingredients:
- ½ head of cauliflower, chopped into small florets
- 1 tablespoon olive oil
- 1 teaspoon Himalayan salt
- 1 teaspoon black pepper, crushed
- 1 tablespoon coconut oil
- ½ cup cooked quinoa
- ¼ cup almonds, chopped
- ½ cup cilantro, chopped
- 1 tablespoon mint, chopped
- ½ cup watercress, chopped

Tahini Dressing
- 3 tablespoons tahini
- 1 tablespoon cashews, soaked overnight
- ¼ teaspoon cumin
- 1 garlic clove
- 1 lemon, juiced
- ¼ cup olive oil
- 1 teaspoon Himalayan salt
- 1 teaspoon black pepper, crushed

Directions:
1. Preheat oven to 425°F/220°C. Place cauliflower on parchment lined baking pan and drizzle with olive oil, salt and pepper. Roast for 15 minutes turning once halfway through.
2. In a food processor, combine all the dressing ingredients and mix until creamy.
3. Heat coconut oil in a skillet. Add quinoa, cooking 5 - 8 minutes or until toasted.
4. In a large bowl add cauliflower, quinoa, almonds, cilantro, mint and watercress. Add in dressing and mix to combine.

---

270 - Stuffed Peppers

Servings: 2
Total Time: 30 minutes

Ingredients:
- 1 cup quinoa, cooked
- ½ cup green lentils, cooked
- 1 small red bell pepper, diced
- 1 small cucumber, diced
- ½ avocado, diced
- 2 tablespoons olive oil
- 1 teaspoon cumin
- 1 teaspoon chili powder
- ½ lime, juiced
- 1 tablespoon cilantro, chopped
- 1 teaspoon salt
- 1 teaspoon black pepper, crushed
- 2 small to medium bell peppers (assorted colors), tops cut off and seeds removed

Directions:
1. In a large bowl, combine the quinoa, lentil, diced bell pepper, cucumber and avocado.
2. Whisk together the olive oil, cumin, chili, lime juice, cilantro, salt and pepper. Pour over quinoa lentil mixture and stir.
3. Stuff each pepper with equal parts of the mixture.

271 - Raw Beetroot Lasagna

Servings: 2
Total Time: 30 minutes

Ingredients:
- ¾ cup cashews, soaked overnight and drained
- 1 teaspoon Himalayan salt
- 1 teaspoon pepper
- 1 teaspoon oregano
- 1 teaspoon dried basil
- ½ lemon, juiced
- 2 zucchinis, sliced thinly with a vegetable peeler

Beetroot Hummus

- 1 small beet, peeled and grated
- 2 cups chickpeas, cooked
- 2 tablespoons tahini
- 1 lemon, juiced
- 1 teaspoon cumin
- 1 teaspoon Himalayan salt

Directions:
1. In a food processor, combine cashews with salt, pepper, oregano, basil and lemon juice until smooth. Set aside and clean the food processor.
2. Combine the beet, chickpeas, tahini, lemon juice, cumin and salt until creamy.
3. In a deep baking dish create a layer of zucchini noodles. Top with Beet Hummus and then cashew mixture. Repeat until all ingredients are used.
4. Chill 15 minutes before serving.

272 - Baba Ganoush Pasta

Servings: 2
Total Time: 35 minutes

Ingredients:
- 6 ounces spelt pasta
- 1 tablespoon olive oil
- 1 eggplant, cubed
- 1 zucchini, cubed
- ½ red bell pepper, cubed
- 1 medium-sized onion, chopped
- 1 garlic clove, minced
- 1 small chili pepper, seeded and chopped
- 1 cup vegetable stock
- 1/2 teaspoon Himalayan salt
- 1 pinch of cayenne pepper
- ¼ cup parsley, chopped

Directions:
1. Cook pasta according to package directions. Set aside.
2. Heat olive oil in a skillet and add eggplant, zucchini, pepper, onion, garlic and chili pepper. Cook for 5 - 8 minutes.
3. Add vegetable stock and let cook another 3 - 5 minutes. Let cool before adding to blender and mixing until smooth.
4. Return sauce back to skillet, season with salt and cayenne pepper. Toss in cooked pasta, sprinkle parsley and serve.

273 - "Cheesy" Broccoli Bowl

Servings: 2
Total Time: 15 minutes

Ingredients:
- 1 teaspoon olive oil
- 1 cup quinoa, cooked
- 4 cups broccoli florets, cooked
- 1 tablespoon lemon juice
- ¼ cup nutritional yeast
- ½ teaspoon Himalayan salt
- ½ teaspoon black pepper, crushed

Directions:
1. In a skillet over medium heat add olive oil, cooked quinoa and broccoli. Cook for 5 minutes or until warmed.
2. Stir in lemon juice, nutritional yeast, salt and pepper.
3. Remove from heat and serve warm.

274 - Lentil & Green Bean Pesto Salad

Servings: 2
Total Time: 20 minutes

Ingredients:
- 2 cups green lentils, cooked
- 1 cup cherry tomatoes, halved
- 2 cups green beans, sliced into 1 inch pieces
- ¼ cup apple cider vinegar
- 2 tablespoons scallion (optional)

Pesto Sauce
- ¾ cup fresh basil leaves
- ½ cup spinach
- 2 tablespoons pine nuts
- 1 garlic clove, chopped
- ¼ cup olive oil
- 1 teaspoon Himalayan salt

Directions:
1. Combine Pesto ingredients in a food processor or blender until smooth and creamy.
2. In a large bowl combine lentils, tomatoes, green beans, vinegar and scallions.
3. Drizzle Pesto Sauce over the lentil mixture and toss well to coat before serving.

275 - Vegetable Packed Minestrone

Servings: 2
Total Time: 20 minutes

Ingredients:
- 1 tablespoon olive oil
- ½ cup of eggplant, cubed
- ½ cup of butternut squash, cubed
- ½ cup of zucchini, cubed
- ½ cup of carrot, diced
- 1 shallot
- 1 garlic clove, minced
- ½ cup kidney beans
- 1 cup of vegetable stock
- 1 cup of diced tomatoes
- 1 tablespoon oregano
- 2 teaspoons Himalayan salt
- 1 teaspoon black pepper
- 1 cup fresh basil
- 1 cup spinach

Directions:
1. In stock pot heat olive oil and add eggplant, squash, zucchini, carrot, shallot and garlic. Cook for 5 minutes, stirring occasionally.
2. To the pot, add kidney beans, stock, diced tomatoes, oregano, salt and black pepper. Simmer another 10 minutes and season more to taste.
3. Before serving, stir in basil and spinach.

276 - Noodle Soup with Greens

Servings: 2
Total Time: 20 minutes

Ingredients:
- 4 ounces soba noodles
- 2 cups water
- 1 ½ tablespoons coconut aminos
- 1 teaspoon ginger, grated
- ½ garlic clove, grated
- ¼ teaspoon Himalayan salt
- ½ cup shelled edamame beans
- ½ cup mushrooms, sliced
- ½ cup green peas
- ½ red bell pepper, sliced thin
- 1 ½ cups chopped baby bok choy - use both stems and greens

Directions:
1. Cook soba noodles according to package directions.
2. In a large stock pot, add water, aminos, ginger, garlic, salt, edamame, mushrooms, peas and bell pepper. Cook 15 minutes over medium low heat.
3. Just before serving, stir in bok choy and cook 1 minute.
4. Divide vegetables, broth and noodles evenly amongst two bowls.

277 - Southwest Tofu Burger

Servings: 2
Total Time: 50 minutes

Ingredients:
- 1 tablespoon olive oil
- ½ yellow onion, diced
- 1 cup green bell pepper, diced
- 1 carrot, diced
- 1 teaspoon Himalayan salt
- 1 teaspoon ground cumin
- ½ teaspoon ground cayenne pepper
- ½ teaspoon black pepper, crushed
- 4 ounces firm tofu, pressed between two heavy plates for at least 30 minutes
- 1 tablespoon nutritional yeast
- 1 tablespoon walnuts, finely crushed
- 1 tablespoon Dijon mustard
- 1 cup arugula
- 2 Bibb lettuce leaves
- 1 avocado, sliced

Directions:
1. Heat olive oil in a medium skillet over medium-low heat. Add onion, bell pepper, carrot, salt, cumin, cayenne and black pepper. Cook for 5 - 8 minutes or until vegetables are soft.
2. Place vegetables in a bowl and let cool for 5 minutes. Discard liquid from the pressed tofu and grate tofu over the bowl. Add nutritional yeast, walnuts and Dijon mustard. Combine well until the mixture can be shaped into 2 burgers.
3. Preheat oven to 400°F/205°C. Place burgers on a baking tray lined with parchment paper. Bake for 30 minutes or until browned.
4. Allow to cool for 5 minutes then divide arugula between the lettuce leaves, top each with a burger and the sliced avocado.

278 - Zucchini Rolls with Red Sauce

Servings: 2
Total Time: 50 minutes

Ingredients:
- 1 tablespoon olive oil
- 1 yellow onion, finely chopped
- 3 Roma tomatoes, finely diced
- 1 red bell pepper, finely diced
- 1 teaspoon Himalayan salt
- 1 teaspoon dried oregano
- ¾ cup water
- 2 medium zucchinis, sliced into thin ribbons with a vegetable peeler
- 10 - 15 fresh basil leaves

Cashew Basil Filling

- 1 cup cashews, soaked overnight and drained
- 1 lemon, juiced
- 3 tablespoons water
- 1 tablespoon nutritional yeast
- ½ teaspoon Himalayan salt
- ¼ teaspoon black pepper, crushed
- ¼ teaspoon ground nutmeg
- 1 handful fresh basil, roughly chopped

Directions:
1. Heat oil in a medium skillet over medium heat. Add onion, tomato, bell pepper, salt and oregano to form the "red veggie mixture". Cook for 8 minutes or until vegetables are soft. Add water and let simmer for another 10 minutes. Transfer cooled vegetable mixture to food processor and blend until smooth.
2. Place ingredients for the Cashew Basil Filling in the cleaned food processor and blend until smooth. This may take up to 10 minutes and you may need to add additional water to thin it out.
3. Place zucchini ribbons on a platter in front of you and divide the Cashew Basil Filling amongst each ribbon. Roll up each zucchini ribbon tightly and place in a glass baking dish which has a light layer of the red veggie mixture spread on the bottom.
4. Top each of the rolls with the remaining red veggie mixture and cook for 15 minutes in an oven that has been preheated to 375°F/190°C. Remove from oven and top each roll with fresh basil leaf.

279 - Lentil, Walnut & Arugula Salad

Servings: 2
Total Time: 20 minutes

Ingredients:

- 1 cup green lentils, cooked & drained
- 1 beet, roasted, peeled and diced
- ½ cup walnuts, toasted and chopped
- 2 cups arugula
- 2 teaspoons lemon zest

Mustard Dressing

- 1 tablespoon olive oil
- 1 tablespoon lemon juice
- 1 tablespoon Dijon mustard
- ¼ teaspoon salt
- ¼ teaspoon pepper

Directions:

1. In a large bowl combine lentils, beets, walnuts, arugula and lemon zest. Set aside
2. Combine Dijon mustard and lemon juice in a small bowl. Slowly whisk in olive oil. Season with salt and pepper
3. Pour Mustard Dressing over lentil salad and combine. Let sit at least 10 minutes before serving.

---

280 - Meatless Taco Wraps

Servings: 2
Total Time: 20 minutes

Ingredients:

- 1 ½ cups brown lentils, cooked
- ½ cup walnuts, toasted
- 1 tablespoon tomato paste
- 1 garlic clove, minced
- ½ teaspoon smoked paprika
- ½ teaspoon chili powder
- ½ teaspoon cumin
- ½ teaspoon Himalayan salt
- ¼ cup water
- 4 romaine leaves
- ½ avocado, sliced

Rainbow Salsa

- ½ cup mango, diced
- ½ cup red bell pepper, diced
- ½ cup green bell pepper, diced
- 3 tablespoons cilantro, chopped
- 1 tablespoon apple cider vinegar
- ½ teaspoon Himalayan salt
- ½ teaspoon black pepper, crushed

Directions:

1. Make Rainbow Salsa by placing all Rainbow Salsa ingredients in a medium bowl and stirring to combine. Let sit for 10 minutes while you make the taco meat.
2. In a food processor, pulse together the lentils, walnuts, tomato paste, garlic, paprika, chili powder, cumin, salt and water. The mixture should be crumbly and not overly smooth.
3. Place the lentil & walnut mixture into each of the romaine leaves and top with Rainbow Salsa and avocado slices.

281 - Quinoa & Black Sesame Pilaf

Servings: 2
Total Time: 25 minutes

Ingredients:
- 1 cup green beans, trimmed and cut into 1 inch pieces
- 2 carrots, peeled and sliced into matchsticks
- 2 tablespoons olive oil, divided
- 2 teaspoons Himalayan salt, divided
- 2 teaspoons black pepper, crushed and divided
- 1 shallot, sliced
- 1 celery stalk, finely diced
- ½ cup green bell pepper, finely diced
- 1 garlic clove, minced
- ½ cup quinoa
- 1 cup vegetable broth or water
- 1 cup green lentils, cooked

Dressing
- 1/3 cup avocado oil
- 2 teaspoons toasted sesame oil
- 1 teaspoon fresh ginger, grated
- 1 teaspoon lemon zest
- ½ teaspoon red chili flakes
- ¼ cup tamari
- ¼ cup rice vinegar
- 2 tablespoons black sesame seeds, toasted

Directions:
1. Place green beans and carrots on a parchment paper lined baking tray and drizzle with 1 tablespoon of olive oil, 1 teaspoon salt and 1 teaspoon black pepper. Cook under the broiler for about 5 minutes or until browned, turning about halfway through.
2. In a large pot, add remaining 1 tablespoon olive oil, shallot, celery, bell pepper and garlic, cooking for 5 minutes. Add quinoa, stirring to coat and cook 2 minutes, until toasted. Add broth or water, bring to a boil and then reduce heat and let simmer for 5 - 8 minutes or until liquid is absorbed.
3. To make dressing, add all dressing ingredients to a bowl and whisk to combine.
4. To assemble, mix together the lentils and quinoa. Season with remaining 1 teaspoon salt and 1 teaspoon pepper. Top with green bean and carrot mixture before drizzling dressing over entire dish.

282 - Lemon Zucchini Pasta

Servings: 2
Total Time: 15 minutes

Ingredients:
- 4 zucchinis
- 2 cups baby spinach, roughly chopped
- 1 cup kale, stems removed and roughly chopped
- ¼ cup fresh basil
- ¼ cup parsley
- 3 garlic cloves
- 1 lemon, juiced
- ¼ cup cashews, soaked overnight and drained
- 2 teaspoons red chili flakes
- 2 teaspoons lemon zest
- 1 cup olive oil
- 1 teaspoon Himalayan salt
- 1 teaspoon black pepper, crushed
- ½ cup cherry tomatoes, sliced in half
- ¼ cup pine nuts, toasted

Directions:
1. Using a spiralizer (or a vegetable peeler to make wider noodles), make zucchini into noodles and set aside.
2. In a food processor combine the spinach, kale, basil, parsley, garlic, lemon juice, cashews, red chili flakes and lemon zest. Once finely chopped, slowly drizzle in olive oil.
3. In a large bowl, toss together the zucchini noodles with the spinach/kale sauce. Season with salt and pepper before garnishing with tomatoes and pine nuts.

283 - Sweet Potato Stew

Servings: 2
Total Time: 50 minutes

Ingredients:
- 1 tablespoon olive oil
- ½ yellow onion, diced
- 2 garlic cloves, minced
- 1 tablespoon tomato paste
- 1 tablespoon apple cider vinegar
- ¼ cup rice flour
- 2 cups vegetable broth
- 1 tablespoon tamari
- 1 tablespoon coconut aminos
- 1 large carrot, cut into 1 inch pieces
- 1 cup sweet potatoes, cut into 1 inch chunks
- 1 stalk of celery, cut into ½ inch pieces
- 1 cup green peas, defrosted if frozen
- ½ tomato, diced
- 1 bay leaf
- 1 teaspoon black pepper
- 1 teaspoon dried thyme
- 1 teaspoon oregano
- ¼ cup parsley, chopped

Directions:
1. Heat oil in a large pot over medium heat. Add onion and garlic and cook for 5 minutes. Add tomato paste, vinegar and rice flour. Stir the mixture with a spoon consistently for 5 more minutes.
2. Pour in broth, tamari and aminos and add carrot, sweet potato, celery, peas, tomato, bay leaf, pepper, thyme and oregano.
3. Let come to a boil and then reduce heat to low and simmer for 20 minutes.
4. After 10 minutes, stir in parsley and serve.

284 - Cashew Zoodles

Servings: 2
Total Time: 30 minutes

Ingredients:
- 1 small zucchini, cut into noodles with a spiralizer
- 1 yellow squash, cut into noodles with a spiralizer
- 1 ¼ teaspoon Himalayan salt
- 2 cups cashews, soaked overnight and drained
- 1 lemon, juiced
- 3 tablespoons water
- 2 tablespoons olive oil
- ¼ teaspoon turmeric
- 1 garlic clove
- 1 teaspoon onion powder
- 2 tablespoons nutritional yeast
- 1 teaspoon black pepper
- 10 cherry tomatoes, halved
- 2 teaspoons chives

Directions:
1. Place zucchini and squash noodles in a colander in the sink and sprinkle with ¼ teaspoon salt. Let sit for at least 2o minutes before rinsing the noodles and letting dry briefly.
2. Add the cashews, lemon juice, water, olive oil, turmeric, garlic, onion powder, nutritional yeast, 1 teaspoon salt and pepper to a blender or food processor. Blend until smooth, adding more water if necessary.
3. In a serving bowl combine the noodles, cherry tomatoes and the cashew mixture. Garnish with chives.

285 - Butternut Squash Risotto

Servings: 2
Total Time: 1 hour 10 minutes

Ingredients:
- 1 cup butternut squash, peeled, seeded and cut into small cubes
- 1 teaspoon olive oil
- 3 cups vegetable broth
- 1 tablespoon ghee
- ½ yellow onion, diced
- ½ bunch kale, stems removed and cut into thin ribbons
- 4 fresh sage leaves, thinly sliced
- ½ teaspoon Himalayan pink salt
- ¼ teaspoon freshly ground pepper
- ½ cup brown rice
- 1 cup butternut squash, peeled, seeded and cut into small cubes
- 1 cup brown rice
- 1 tablespoon chives, thinly sliced

Directions:
1. Roast butternut squash in an oven preheated to 400°F/205°C by lining squash cubes on a baking tray lined with parchment paper and drizzling squash with 1 teaspoon olive oil. Roast for 25 minutes, flipping once.
2. In a small saucepan, bring broth to a low simmer over low heat.
3. Place ghee in a large saucepan over medium-low heat and add onion, kale, sage salt and pepper. Cook 5 minutes before adding brown rice and cooking another 2 minutes to toast.
4. Add butternut squash and brown rice to the large saucepan before adding a ¼ cup of the broth and stirring. Reduce heat to low. Continue adding ¼ cup broth and stirring once the previously adding liquid has been absorbed. This may take up to 50 minutes.
5. Remove risotto and place in serving bowl and garnish with chives.

286 - Meatless Meatloaf Cups

Servings: 2 (3 cups per serving)
Total Time: 1 hour 10 minutes

Ingredients:
- 1 tablespoon of ground flaxseeds + 3 ½ tablespoons of water
- 1 ½ tablespoon olive oil
- 1 small carrot, peeled and cut into 1 inch pieces
- 1 small celery stalk, cut into 1 inch pieces
- 1 shallot, diced
- 1 garlic clove, minced
- ½ cup button mushrooms, diced
- 1 cup brown lentils, cooked
- ¼ cup walnuts, toasted
- ½ cup almond meal
- 1 teaspoon Dijon mustard
- 1 teaspoon paprika
- 1 teaspoon Himalayan salt
- 1 teaspoon black pepper
- ½ tablespoon olive oil
- 1 tablespoon tomato paste
- 1 teaspoon raw honey
- 1 teaspoon coconut aminos
- 1 teaspoon tamari

Directions:
1. In a small bowl, whisk to combine the flaxseeds and water. Set aside.
2. Heat 1 tablespoon olive oil in a medium skillet over medium-low heat. Add carrot, celery, shallots and garlic. Cook 10 minutes, stirring frequently. Add mushrooms and cook another 10 minutes.
3. Place lentils and walnuts in food processor and pulse together about 10 times. Add vegetable mixture to the food processor and mix until combined but not entirely smooth. Add mixture to a bowl and fold in the almond meal, flaxseeds mixture, mustard, paprika, salt and pepper.
4. Lightly grease 6 places in a muffin tin with ½ tablespoon olive oil. Add lentil and vegetable mixture to each and press to mold.
5. In a small bowl, combine tomato paste, honey, coconut aminos and tamari. Brush tomato mixture on top of each meatloaf cup.
6. Bake in an oven that has been preheated to 350°F/180°C for 40 minutes. Tops should be lightly browned when finished.

287 - Spicy Dal & Greens

Servings: 2
Total Time: 30 minutes

Ingredients:
- 1 tablespoon ghee
- 1 jalapeno, seeded and diced
- ¼ teaspoon ground cumin
- ¼ teaspoon turmeric
- ¼ teaspoon ground cardamom
- ⅛ teaspoon ground fenugreek
- 1 inch piece ginger, grated
- 1 garlic clove, minced
- 1 small onion, diced
- 1 small tomato, diced
- ½ cup red lentils, rinsed and drained
- 1 cup vegetable broth
- ¼ teaspoon Himalayan salt
- 1 teaspoon black pepper, crushed
- 2 tablespoons cilantro, chopped
- 1 lime, zest

Directions:
1. Heat ghee in a medium saucepan over medium high heat. Add jalapeno, cumin, turmeric, cardamom, fenugreek, ginger, garlic and onion. Cook 5 minutes and then add tomato and red lentils. Stir and cook for an additional minute.
2. Pour vegetable broth into the saucepan and add salt and pepper. Bring to a boil and then reduce heat to low and simmer about 15 - 20 minutes or until lentils are soft.
3. Garnish with cilantro and lime zest.

288 - Blackened Salmon with Fruit Salsa

Servings: 2
Total Time: 20 minutes

Ingredients:
- 8 ounces wild salmon fillet, skin-on
- 1 teaspoon cayenne pepper
- 1 teaspoon garlic powder
- ½ teaspoon chili powder
- ¼ teaspoon Himalayan salt
- ¼ teaspoon black pepper, crushed
- 1 tablespoon olive oil
- 4 cups mixed greens (e.g. spring onions, broccoli, spinach)

Mango Pineapple Salsa

- ½ green bell pepper, seeded and diced into small pieces
- ½ cup mango, diced into small pieces
- ½ cup pineapple, diced into small pieces
- 1 lime, zested and juiced
- 1 tablespoon cilantro, finely chopped
- Pinch Himalayan salt

Directions:
1. Make the Mango Pineapple Salsa by placing all the Mango Pineapple Salsa ingredients in a small bowl and combining well. Set aside.
2. In a small bowl, combine the cayenne, garlic powder, chili powder, salt and pepper. Place mixture on flat plate.
3. Heat a cast iron skillet on the stovetop over medium heat. Brush the olive oil on each side of each fillet and then place the flesh side in the spice mixture on the plate.
4. Place the fish, flesh side down in the pan and cook about 5 minutes. Flip over cook an additional 6 minutes or until fish is done.
5. Serve fish over mixed greens (of your liking) and spoon salsa on top.

289 - Roasted Cauliflower with Chimichurri Sauce

Servings: 2
Total Time: 40 minutes

Ingredients:
- 1 small head cauliflower (about 1 pound), stem removed
- 2 tablespoons avocado oil, divided
- 1 teaspoon Himalayan salt, divided
- 1 teaspoon dried oregano
- ½ teaspoon black pepper
- 2 garlic cloves, minced and divided
- 3 cups green beans, trimmed
- 15 cherry tomatoes, halved
- 1 teaspoon lemon zest

Chimichurri Sauce

- ¼ cup apple cider vinegar
- ½ teaspoon Himalayan salt
- 2 garlic cloves
- 1 shallot, sliced
- 1 teaspoon red chili flakes
- 1 teaspoon fresh oregano (or dried)
- ¼ cup cilantro, chopped
- ¼ cup flat-leaf parsley, chopped
- 1/3 cup olive oil

Directions:
1. Make Chimichurri Sauce by placing all ingredients except the olive oil in a food processor or blender and blend until combined. While the food processor is running, drizzle in the olive oil. Let it sit while preparing the cauliflower.
2. Slice the cauliflower in half lengthwise and cut two steaks from each side of the core (saving any leftover cauliflower that falls loose).
3. Heat a large cast iron skillet (or ovenproof skillet) on the stove over medium-high heat. Add 1 tablespoon of the avocado oil and once heated, place cauliflower steaks into the skillet. Season with 1/4 teaspoon salt, ½ teaspoon oregano and ¼ teaspoon black pepper. After 4 minutes, flip and season the other side with ¼ teaspoon salt, ½ teaspoon oregano and ¼ teaspoon black pepper. Cook for another 4 minutes before placing pan in an oven that has been preheated to 400°F/205°C. Roast for 20 minutes or until cauliflower is tender.
4. On a baking tray lined with parchment paper, place the green beans and tomatoes. Drizzle with remaining olive oil and sprinkle salt, pepper, garlic and lemon zest on top. Roast in the oven with the cauliflower for 15 minutes, turning once.
5. Serve cauliflower on top of the green bean/tomato mixture and drizzled with Chimichurri Sauce.

290 - Cook-off Chili

Servings: 2
Total Time: 20 minutes

Ingredients:
- 1 tablespoon olive oil
- ½ small onion, diced
- 1 jalapeno pepper, seeded and diced
- 1 small carrot, diced
- ½ red bell pepper, seeded and diced
- 1 small tomato, diced
- 1 tablespoon tomato paste
- 2 garlic cloves, minced
- 1 ½ teaspoon chili powder
- 1 ½ teaspoon cumin powder
- ½ cup cooked red beans
- ½ cup quinoa, cooked
- 2 cups vegetable stock
- 1 lime, sliced in half
- 2 tablespoons cilantro, chopped
- 2 tablespoons unsweetened yogurt

Directions:
1. In a large pot over medium heat, add olive oil, onion, jalapeno, carrot and red bell pepper. Cook 8 minutes or until softened. Add in tomatoes, tomato paste, garlic, chili powder, cumin, red beans, quinoa and vegetable stock.
2. Bring to a boil, reduce heat to low and simmer 15 minutes.
3. Serve in two bowls and garnish each bowl with ½ lime, 1 tablespoon cilantro and 1 tablespoon yogurt each.

291 - Pasta & Veggie Stroganoff

Servings: 2
Total Time: 20 minutes

Ingredients:
- 8 ounces gluten-free pasta
- 1 tablespoon olive oil
- 1 garlic clove, minced
- 1 cup mushrooms, sliced
- 2 cups spinach
- 1 teaspoon red pepper flakes
- 1 teaspoon oregano
- ½ teaspoon nutmeg
- 1 cup unsweetened almond milk
- 1 cup vegetable broth
- 1 teaspoon arrowroot starch
- ¼ teaspoon Himalayan salt
- ½ teaspoon black pepper, crushed
- ¼ cup parsley, chopped

Directions:
1. Cook pasta according to package directions.
2. In a large skillet over medium heat, add olive oil, garlic and mushrooms. Cook 5 minutes then add spinach, red pepper, oregano, nutmeg and cook 3 more minutes.
3. Pour in almond milk and vegetable broth. Sprinkle the arrowroot starch on top and stir well. Let come to a low boil then reduce heat to a simmer and cook 5 minutes. Season with salt and pepper.
4. Place pasta on a plate and top with mushroom spinach mixture. Garnish with chopped parsley.

292 - Tofu Mole with Jicama Salad

Servings: 2
Total Time: 35 minutes

Ingredients:
- 4 cups kale, stems removed and sliced into thin ribbons
- 1 tablespoon olive oil
- 1 lemon, juiced
- ½ teaspoon Himalayan salt
- 8 ounces firm tofu, cubed and baked
- 1 cup jicama, peeled and shredded
- 1 tablespoon raisins
- 1 teaspoon slivered almonds

Mole Sauce

- 1 tablespoon olive oil
- ½ onion, chopped
- 1 garlic clove, minced
- 1/3 cup slivered almonds
- ¼ cup raisins
- 3 dates, pitted, soaked 15 minutes and drained
- ½ teaspoon Himalayan salt
- ¼ teaspoon cinnamon
- ½ teaspoon ground coriander
- 1 teaspoon cumin
- 1 teaspoon dried thyme
- 1 teaspoon chili powder
- ¼ teaspoon ground cloves
- 1 teaspoon chipotle in adobo sauce
- 1 tablespoon tomato paste
- ¼ cup diced tomatoes
- ½ cup water
- 1 tablespoon raw cacao

Directions:
1. Place kale in a large bowl and add in olive oil. Massage gently then add lemon juice and salt. Set aside while making Mole Sauce.
2. Make Mole Sauce by heating olive oil in a large saucepan over medium heat. Add the onion, garlic, almonds, raisins and dates. Cook for 8 minutes. Stir in the salt, cinnamon, coriander, cumin, thyme, chili powder and cloves. Cook 1 minute.
3. Add chipotle, tomato paste, tomatoes, water and cacao to the saucepan and simmer for 15 minutes. Turn heat off and blend with immersion blender (or let cool and blend in a blender).
4. Add Mole Sauce back to the saucepan and add baked tofu. Turn heat to low and allow to heat through.
5. Toss jicama, raisins and almonds in the kale mixture and place on a plate along with the tofu mole.

293 - Green Pea Pasta

Servings: 2
Total Time: 35 minutes

Ingredients:
- ½ tablespoon olive oil
- 1 garlic clove, minced
- 1 ½ tablespoons ginger, peeled and grated
- 2 cups spinach
- 1 cup coconut milk
- 1 tablespoon lime juice
- ½ teaspoon red chili flakes
- ½ cup cilantro
- ½ cup green peas, defrosted
- 2 medium zucchinis, spiralized into noodles
- 1 teaspoon Himalayan salt
- 1 teaspoon black pepper

Directions:
1. Heat oil in a medium skillet over medium heat. Add garlic and ginger and cook 3 minutes. Add spinach, coconut milk, lime juice, chili flakes and cilantro. Simmer for 5 minutes.
2. Add mixture to a high speed blender along with ¼ cup green peas. Blend until smooth to create the saucy mixture.
3. Place medium skillet back over medium heat and add zucchini noodles, remaining ¼ cup peas and sauce. Heat for 3 minutes and sprinkle salt and pepper before serving.

294 - Tricolor Pasta

Servings: 2
Total Time: 20 minutes

Ingredients:
- 2 medium beets, spiralized into noodles
- 1 tablespoon olive oil
- ½ teaspoon Himalayan salt
- ¼ teaspoon black pepper, crushed
- 1 large clove
- 1 teaspoon cayenne

Green Sauce

- 1 cup basil leaves, packed
- 1 cup parsley, chopped
- ½ cup spinach, chopped
- 3 tablespoons almonds
- 1 tablespoon green onion, chopped
- ¼ cup of olive oil
- ½ teaspoon Himalayan salt

Spicy Orange Garnish

- 1 small carrot, shredded
- 1 tablespoon olive oil
- 1 teaspoon red chili flakes
- 1 teaspoon pumpkin seeds, toasted
- ¼ teaspoon turmeric
- 1 teaspoon lemon juice

Directions:
1. Line a baking tray with parchment paper. Coat beet noodles with tablespoon of olive oil and spread on the baking tray. Season with ½ teaspoon salt.
2. Bake in an oven preheated to 400°F/205°C for 15 minutes.
3. In a small bowl, combine ingredients for the Spicy Orange Garnish and set aside.
4. In a food processor or blender, combine all the Green Sauce ingredients and mix until smooth.
5. Remove beet noodles from oven, place in a large bowl and toss with Green Sauce. Top with Spicy Orange Garnish.

295 - Cauliflower Pasta Pillows in Red Sauce

Servings: 2
Total Time: 45 minutes

Ingredients:

- 1 head of cauliflower, steamed
- 1 garlic clove, minced
- 1 cup almond meal of enough to make a soft dough
- ¼ cup arrowroot powder (plus extra for rolling out dough)
- 1 tablespoon ground flaxseeds
- 3 tablespoons water
- 1 tablespoon olive oil
- ½ cup basil leaves, thinly sliced

Red Sauce

- ½ onion, chopped
- 1 tablespoon olive oil
- 1 garlic clove, minced
- 1 small carrot, chopped
- 1 red bell pepper, chopped
- 1 cup cherry tomatoes, halved
- 1 ½ cups vegetable stock
- 1 teaspoon oregano
- 1 teaspoon dried basil
- 1 teaspoon Himalayan salt
- 1 teaspoon pepper

Directions:

1. Whisk together the flaxseeds and water together in a small bowl. Set aside.
2. *For creation of the Red Sauce* In a medium skillet over medium heat, add onion, olive oil, garlic, carrot and red pepper. Cook 10 minutes and then add tomatoes, vegetable stock, oregano, dried basil, salt and pepper. Cook another 10 minutes.
3. Using an immersion blender, blend the Red Sauce until smooth. Reduce heat to low and simmer another 20 minutes while you make the cauliflower pasta.
4. In a food processor, add the cauliflower and garlic. Process until smooth. In a small bowl combine the almond meal, arrowroot powder and flaxseeds mixture (it should now be a gel). Add to the food processor in small increments, blending between each addition. If needed, add some water to make a soft dough.
5. Dust cutting board with extra arrowroot powder and place dough on the board. Roll the dough into 4 equal sized ropes. Cut the ropes into 1 inch pieces. Press each piece lightly with a fork.
6. In a medium skillet, heat olive oil over medium-low heat. Add cauliflower pasta pieces, making sure not to crowd the pan and cook 3 minutes each side.
7. Place cauliflower pasta on a place and top with Red Sauce and basil leaves.

296 - Raw Thai Curry

Servings: 2
Total Time: 10 minutes

Ingredients:

- 2 medium yellow squash, spiralized into noodles
- ½ cup alfalfa sprouts
- ¼ cup green peas, defrosted
- 1 red pepper, sliced
- ¼ red cabbage, shredded
- ¼ cup cilantro, chopped
- 2 tablespoons cashews, toasted and crushed
- 2 tablespoons green onions, thinly sliced

Curry Sauce

- 1 tablespoon green curry paste
- ½ cup raw cashew nuts, soaked for 30 minutes and drained
- ¼ cup water
- ½ lime, juiced
- 2 tablespoons cilantro, chopped
- ¼ cup green onion, chopped
- ¼ cup coconut milk
- ½ teaspoon ground cumin
- ½ teaspoon ground ginger
- 1 garlic clove, minced
- ½ inch piece fresh ginger, grated
- ½ teaspoon ground coriander
- 1 teaspoon red chili flakes

Directions:

1. In a high speed blender, add Curry Sauce ingredients and blend until smooth.
2. Toss together the squash, sprouts, green peas, bell pepper, cabbage and cilantro. Add Curry Sauce and toss to coat well. Garnish with cashews and green onions.

297 - Shrimp & Arugula Salad

Servings: 2
Total Time: 25 minutes

Ingredients:
- 10 large shrimp, peeled, cleaned and deveined
- ½ lemon, juiced
- 2 tablespoons olive oil
- 1 garlic clove, minced
- 1 tablespoon parsley, chopped
- ½ teaspoon Himalayan salt
- ½ teaspoon black pepper, crushed

Arugula Salad

- 4 cups arugula
- 10 cherry tomatoes, halved
- 2 tablespoons apple cider vinegar
- ½ lemon, juiced
- 2 tablespoons olive oil
- 1 teaspoon Himalayan salt
- 2 teaspoons pine nuts, toasted

Directions:
1. In a medium bowl, place shrimp, lemon juice, olive oil, garlic, parsley, salt and pepper. Let sit in the fridge for 15 minutes.
2. Heat a medium skillet or grill pan over medium-high heat. Place shrimp in the skillet and cook 3 minutes each side or until shrimp are pink and firm.
3. Combine the ingredients for the Arugula Salad in a large bowl. Place shrimp on top of the salad and serve.

298 - Avocado and Tomato Pizza

Servings: 2
Total Time: 15 minutes plus 12 hours dehydrating time

Ingredients:
- 1 avocado, sliced
- 1 small tomato, sliced
- 1 cup arugula
- 2 teaspoons olive oil
- 2 tablespoons nutritional yeast
- 1 teaspoon Himalayan salt
- 1 teaspoon lemon juice

Pizza Dough

- 1 ¼ cups sunflower seeds, soaked overnight and drained
- 1/3 cup flaxseeds, ground to a very fine powder
- 1 garlic clove, minced
- 4 tablespoons olive oil
- 1 teaspoon Himalayan salt
- 1 teaspoon black pepper, crushed
- 1 teaspoon dried oregano
- 1 teaspoon dried basil

Directions:
1. In a blender, pulse the drained sunflower seeds a few times then add sunflower mix to a medium bowl along with the flaxseeds flour, garlic, olive oil, salt, pepper, oregano and basil.
2. Knead together the mixture until a dough forms (add a little water if needed). Roll out dough into a pizza shape and place on a baking tray lined with parchment paper.
3. Heat oven to lowest possible temperature. Place baking tray in the oven and dehydrate in the oven for at least 12 hours.
4. When Pizza Dough is ready, layer avocado and tomato slices on top of the crust. Toss arugula in a small bowl with olive oil, nutritional yeast, salt and lemon juice. Place arugula on top of avocado and tomato. Serve immediately.

299 - Spinach Ravioli

Servings: 2
Total Time: 1 hour

Ingredients:

- 1 tablespoon flaxseed, ground
- 6 tablespoons water, divided
- 1 cup spelt flour
- 1 teaspoon Himalayan salt

Spinach Filling

- 1 tablespoon flaxseed, ground
- 3 tablespoons water
- ½ cup mushrooms, sliced
- 1 cup spinach
- 1 teaspoon olive oil
- 1 tablespoon parsley, chopped
- 1 tablespoon nutritional yeast

Simple Red Sauce

- 1 cup cherry tomatoes, halved
- 1 red bell pepper, chopped
- 2 tablespoons olive oil
- 1 clove garlic, grated
- ½ cup water
- 1 teaspoon oregano
- 1 teaspoon Himalayan salt
- 1 teaspoon pepper

Directions:

1. Make the spinach filling by whisking together the ground flaxseeds and water together in a small bowl and letting sit for 15 minutes. After 15 minutes, add flax mixture and remaining Spinach Filling ingredients to a food processor and combine. Set aside.
2. Prepare Simple Red Sauce by combining all Simple Red Sauce ingredients in a blender and combining until smooth.
3. To make ravioli, begin by creating a flask egg by whisking together 1 tablespoon flaxseeds with 3 tablespoons water and letting rest 15 minutes. When ready, combine flax mixture, spelt flour, salt and remaining 3 tablespoons water in a food processor until a dough forms. Let dough rest for 20 minutes.
4. Roll out dough and use a ravioli maker to fill each with the Spinach Filling and top with second layer of dough. Seal edges with water.
5. Boil water in a medium saucepan and once at a rolling boil, drop in ravioli and cook 6 minutes. Strain and set aside.
6. Add Simple Red Sauce to medium saucepan and bring to a simmer. Add ravioli and cook 2 minutes until warmed.

---

300 - Kale & Squash Vegetable Gratin

Servings: 2
Total Time: 50 minutes

Ingredients:

- 2 tablespoons ghee
- 1 garlic clove, finely minced
- 1 leek, finely chopped
- 1 fennel bulb, sliced
- 2 cups kale, stems removed and thinly sliced
- 2 cups butternut squash, cubed and roasted
- ¼ cup rice flour
- ½ cup unsweetened almond milk, warmed
- 1 teaspoon dried sage
- ½ teaspoon nutmeg
- 1 teaspoon Himalayan salt
- 1 teaspoon black pepper, crushed

Crumb Topping

- 1 ½ tablespoons ghee
- 1 cup gluten-free oats
- ¼ cup almond meal
- ¼ cup almonds, slivered
- 1 teaspoon fresh sage, torn
- 1 teaspoon Himalayan salt

Directions:

1. Prepare vegetable filling by heating 1 tablespoon ghee in a medium saucepan over medium heat. Add garlic, leek and fennel. Cook 10 minutes and then add kale. Cook another 5 minutes and then transfer to a small baking dish. Place roasted butternut squash on top of the vegetable mixture.
2. Make the sauce by adding 1 tablespoon ghee to the medium saucepan and heat over medium-low heat. When ghee is melted, whisk in rice flour and continue to move around the pan about 5 minutes. Pour in warmed almond milk while continuing to whisk. Bring to a boil, then reduce heat to low and simmer. Season with sage, nutmeg, salt and pepper.
3. Pour sauce over the vegetable and squash mixture, making sure it is well combined. Preheat oven to 325°F/170°C.
4. To make the Crumb Topping, melt 1 ½ tablespoons ghee in a large skillet. Then add remaining Crumb Topping ingredients. Let cool slightly and then crumble the mixture on top of the vegetable and squash mixture.
5. Bake in the oven for 30 minutes. Serve immediately from the oven.

301 - Cabbage Rolls

Servings: 2
Total Time: 2 hours 10 minutes

Ingredients:
- ½ cup brown rice, cooked
- 1 celery stalk, finely diced
- 1 carrot, finely diced
- ½ red bell pepper, finely diced
- ½ teaspoon Himalayan salt
- ½ teaspoon garlic powder
- ½ teaspoon onion powder
- 1 teaspoon parsley, chopped
- 2 tablespoons tomato paste
- 4 cups water
- 8 cabbage leaves
- 2 cups vegetable broth

Directions:
1. Prepare vegetable filling combining brown rice, celery, carrots, red bell pepper, salt, garlic powder, onion powder, parsley and tomato paste in a medium bowl. Set aside in the fridge until ready to use.
2. In a large pot, bring 4 cups water to a boil. Add cabbage leaves for 1 minute then turn heat off and let sit, covered, for 1 hour.
3. Remove cabbage leaves from the pot and discard water. Spoon vegetable and rice mixture into each of the cabbage leaves. Roll each cabbage leaf, ensuring there are no openings and secure with a toothpick.
4. Add vegetable broth to the large pot and lay cabbage rolls on the bottom, toothpick side down. Turn heat to low and simmer for 1 hour.

302 - Lentil Stuffed Squash

Servings: 2
Total Time: 30 minutes

Ingredients:
- 1 tablespoon olive oil
- ½ cup red bell pepper, finely diced
- ½ cup zucchini, finely diced
- 1 shallot, diced
- 1 garlic clove, minced
- 2 small acorn squash, halved and seeded
- Non-Stick Vegetable Spray
- ½ cup brown lentils, cooked
- ½ cup quinoa, cooked
- 2 tablespoons coconut aminos

Directions:
1. Preheat oven to 350°F/180°C.
2. In a small skillet over medium heat, add olive oil, bell pepper, zucchini, shallot and garlic. Cook 5 minutes and set aside.
3. Place acorn squash in a medium baking dish sprayed with Non-Stick Vegetable Spray and pour water into the pan so that is ¼ up the side of the squash. Bake 15 minutes and remove.
4. In a small bowl, combine the vegetable mixture, brown lentils, quinoa and coconut aminos.
5. Fill each acorn half with the lentil and vegetable mixture and place back in the oven for 10 minutes.

303 - Pomegranate Pumpkins

Servings: 2
Total Time: 35 minutes

Ingredients:
- 1 small sugar pumpkin, halved and seeds removed
- 1 tablespoon coconut oil, melted
- ½ cup brown rice, cooked
- ½ cup cooked chickpeas, cooked
- 3 tablespoons pomegranate seeds
- 5 tablespoons parsley, finely chopped
- 1 tablespoon chia seeds
- 1 garlic clove, minced
- 1 teaspoon Himalayan salt
- 1 tablespoon lemon juice
- 1 teaspoon orange juice

Directions:
1. Preheat oven to 350°F/180°C.
2. On a baking tray, place sugar pumpkins and brush with coconut oil. Flip over so that pumpkin is facing down and roast for 25-30 minutes, until flesh is tender.
3. Once pumpkin is cooked, remove the flesh and place in a large mixing bowl. Add in rice, chickpeas, pomegranate seeds, parsley, chia seeds, garlic, salt, lemon juice and orange juice.
4. Place mixture back into pumpkin and serve.

304 - Roasted Green Salad

Servings: 2
Total Time: 35 minutes

Ingredients:
- 2 cups brussel sprouts, halved
- 1 teaspoon avocado oil
- ¼ teaspoon Himalayan salt
- ¼ teaspoon ground cumin
- 2 teaspoon avocado oil
- 1 garlic clove, minced
- 1 shallot, sliced
- 1 cup green cabbage, shredded
- 1 teaspoon ground oregano
- 1 lemon, zested and juiced
- 1 teaspoon apple cider vinegar
- ½ cup frozen peas, defrosted
- 2 tablespoons chopped mint
- 2 tablespoons almonds, slivered

Directions:
1. Preheat oven to 350°F/180°C.
2. On a large baking tray, place brussel sprouts, 1 teaspoon avocado oil, salt and cumin. Toss to coat well and roast for 25 minutes.
3. In a large skillet over medium heat add the other teaspoon of avocado oil, the garlic and shallot. Add the cabbage, oregano, lemon zest and juice and cook for 15 minutes.
4. Add vinegar and peas to the skillet along with the roasted brussel sprouts and cook for 5 minutes. Transfer to large bowl and toss with the mint and almonds.

305 - Roasted Green Salad

Servings: 2
Total Time: 1 hour

Ingredients:
- 4 cups vegetable stock
- 3 tablespoons avocado oil
- 2 garlic cloves, finely minced
- 2 large shallots, finely diced
- 1 cup brown rice
- 2 cups baby spinach, finely chopped
- 1 lemon, zested and juiced
- 1 teaspoon Himalayan salt
- 2 teaspoon black pepper, crushed
- 3 tablespoons green onions, sliced
- 1 cup broccoli sprouts

Directions:
1. In a small saucepan, bring vegetable stock to a low simmer over low heat.
2. In a large stockpot over medium-low, add avocado oil, garlic and shallot. Cook for 5 minutes before stirring in the brown rice. Stir brown rice for 2 minutes in the pan so that it does not burn. Reduce heat to low.
3. Add in 1/3 cup of the vegetable stock and stir frequently until the liquid is absorbed. Once liquid is absorbed, add in another 1/3 cup of stock. Continue doing this until all the stock is used and the rice is tender.
4. While risotto is cooking, add spinach, lemon juice and salt to a blender and combine until smooth.
5. When risotto is cooked, stir in the spinach mixture and let cook for 3 minutes (rice should absorb most of the spinach liquid).
6. Stir in lemon zest and black pepper.
7. Garnish with green onions and broccoli sprouts and serve immediately.

306 - Jumbo Stuffed Mushrooms

Servings: 2
Total Time: 30 minutes

Ingredients:
- 2 large Portobello mushrooms
- 2 tablespoons olive oil
- 1 garlic clove, finely minced
- ½ white onion, diced
- ½ cup almonds, slivered and roughly chopped
- 1 cup spinach, chopped
- 2 tablespoons raisins
- ½ teaspoon cinnamon
- ½ teaspoon nutmeg
- 3 tablespoons water
- 3 tablespoons parsley
- 1 teaspoon Himalayan salt
- 1 teaspoon black pepper, crushe

Directions:
1. Preheat oven to 350°F/180°C.
2. On a large baking tray, place mushrooms, stem side up and drizzle with 1 tablespoon olive oil and the garlic. Roast in the oven for 10 minutes.
3. In a large skillet over medium heat add the other tablespoon of olive oil and the onion. Cook for 5 minutes before adding the almonds, spinach, raisins, cinnamon and nutmeg. Let cook for another 4 minutes and then begin adding the water in, one tablespoon at a time and letting the water absorb in between each addition.
4. Stir in parsley, salt and pepper before placing the mixture on each of the mushrooms.
5. Place back in the oven for another 10 minutes.

307 - Raw Zoodles with Tropical Sauce

Servings: 1
Total Time: 5 minutes

Ingredients:
- ½ mango, diced
- ¼ cup pineapple, diced
- 2 tablespoons orange juice
- ½ avocado
- 3 tablespoons green onions, sliced
- 1 garlic clove
- 1 zucchini, spiralized into noodles

Directions:
1. In a blender, combine the mango, pineapple, orange juice, avocado, onions and garlic.
2. Mix sauce with zucchini noodles and serve.

308 - Spaghetti Squash Pasta Boats

Servings: 2
Total Time: 30 minutes

Ingredients:
- 1 spaghetti squash, halved lengthwise and seeds removed
- 2 tablespoons olive oil
- 1 teaspoon Himalayan salt
- 1 teaspoon black pepper, crushed
- 2 garlic cloves, minced
- 5 handfuls kale, stems removed and sliced thinly
- 1 cup of chickpeas, cooked
- ¼ cup raisins
- ¼ cup of walnuts
- 1 avocado, sliced

Directions:
1. Preheat oven to 350°F/180°C.
2. On a large baking tray, brush squash halves with 1 tablespoon olive oil and season with salt and pepper. Place squash cut side down and roast for 25 minutes or until tender.
3. In a large skillet over medium heat add the other tablespoon of olive oil and the garlic. Cook for 2 minutes before adding the kale, chickpeas, raisins and walnuts. Let cook for another 8 minutes.
4. With a fork, loosen the strands of the squash and then pour in the kale and chickpea mixture.
5. Top with avocado slices.

309 - Sweet Potato Chili

Servings: 2
Total Time: 45 minutes

Ingredients:

- 1 tablespoon coconut oil
- 2 garlic cloves, minced
- ½ yellow onion, diced
- ½ inch knob ginger, minced
- 1 tablespoon turmeric
- ½ teaspoon coriander
- ¼ teaspoon cumin
- ¼ teaspoon cinnamon
- 2 small sweet potatoes, chopped into small chunks
- 1 large tomato, diced
- ½ cup red lentils
- ½ cup quinoa
- 1 15-ounce can tomato puree
- 2 cups water
- 1 bunch kale, stems removed and chopped into pieces
- 1 lemon, juiced
- 1 teaspoon Himalayan salt
- 2 tablespoons green onions, sliced
- 1 tablespoon cashews, chopped

Directions:

1. Heat coconut oil in a large pot over medium heat. Add garlic, onion, ginger, turmeric, coriander, cumin and cinnamon. Cook for 5 minutes and then add sweet potato and let cook for another 5 minutes.
2. Stir in diced tomato, red lentils, quinoa, tomato puree and water. Bring to a boil, reduce heat to low and let simmer for 25 minutes.
3. Stir in kale, lemon juice and salt. Let simmer another 5 minutes.
4. Transfer to bowl and garnish with green onions and cashews.

310 - Sweet Potato Cottage Platter

Servings: 2
Total Time: 50 minutes

Ingredients:

- 2 teaspoons olive oil
- 1 yellow onion, chopped small
- 1 garlic clove, minced
- ½ carrot, diced
- 1 celery stalk, diced
- 5 button mushrooms, sliced
- ½ cup green peas
- 2 tomatoes, diced
- 1 teaspoon cumin powder
- ½ teaspoon turmeric powder
- ½ teaspoon cayenne
- 2 teaspoons tamari sauce
- 1 teaspoon coconut aminos
- ¼ cup tomato paste
- 2 tablespoons water
- 2 bay leaves
- 1 teaspoon chives, sliced

Mashed Topping

- 2 sweet potatoes, peeled and chopped
- 2 cups water
- 1 teaspoon Himalayan salt
- 1 teaspoon nutmeg
- ¼ cup unsweetened almond milk

Directions:

1. In a large saucepan over medium heat, add olive oil, onion, garlic, carrot and celery. Cook for 5 minutes and then add the mushrooms, peas, tomatoes, cumin, turmeric, cayenne, tamari, coconut aminos, tomato paste, water and bay leaves.
2. Reduce heat to low and simmer for 15 minutes. Remove bay leaves and pour vegetable mixture into a small glass baking dish.
3. In a medium saucepan, make the Mashed Topping by covering sweet potatoes with water. Bring to a boil and then reduce heat and let simmer for 20 minutes or until sweet potatoes are tender. Drain potatoes and blend in a food processor with salt, nutmeg and almond milk until smooth.
4. Preheat oven to 350°F/180°C. Place mashed sweet potato on top of the vegetable mixture in the baking dish. Smooth out the top with a knife and bake in the oven for 30 minutes.
5. Garnish with the chives and serve warm.

311 - Italian Stuffed Zucchini

Servings: 2
Total Time: 50 minutes

Ingredients:
- 1 cup cherry tomatoes, halved
- 2 cups spinach, chopped
- 1 tablespoon lemon zest
- ½ teaspoon Himalayan salt
- ½ teaspoon black pepper, crushed
- ½ teaspoon red chili flakes
- 1 garlic clove, grated
- 2 teaspoons pine nuts
- 1 tablespoon olive oil, divided
- 2 large zucchinis, split in half lengthwise and seeds removed
- 1 ½ cup basil, sliced thinly

Directions:
1. Preheat oven to 400°F/205°C.
2. In a small bowl, combine the tomatoes, spinach, zest, salt, black pepper, chili flakes, garlic and pine nuts. Drizzle with half of the olive oil and toss to coat well.
3. Stuff each half of the zucchini with the cherry and spinach mixture. Place on baking tray and roast in the oven for 15 minutes.
4. Remove from the oven and drizzle with remaining olive oil and garnish with basil.

312 - Sushi Bowl

Servings: 2
Total Time: 40 minutes

Ingredients:
- ¼ cup tamari
- 2 tablespoons coconut aminos
- 2 teaspoon sesame oil
- 2 tablespoon sesame seeds
- 2 tablespoon chopped shallots
- 1 garlic clove, minced
- 1 ½ inch piece of ginger, grated
- 1 lime, zested and juiced
- 1 jalapeno, seeded and diced
- 2 sashimi grade tuna medallions, cubed
- 1 cup quinoa, cooked
- 2 tablespoons green onions, sliced
- 3 tablespoons cilantro, chopped
- 1 carrot, spiralized
- 1 avocado

Directions:
1. In a medium sized bowl, whisk the tamari, coconut aminos, 1 teaspoon sesame oil, 1 tablespoon sesame seeds, shallots, garlic, ginger, lime zest, lime juice and jalapeno. Place tuna in the bowl and toss to coat. Place in fridge for 30 minutes.
2. In a separate medium bowl, combine the quinoa, green onions and 1 tablespoon of the cilantro. Place in serving bowls and add spiralized carrot and avocado on one side of each bowl.
3. Remove tuna from fridge and place next to the carrot and avocado. Garnish with 2 tablespoons cilantro, 1 tablespoon sesame seeds and drizzle with 1 teaspoon sesame oil.

313 - Omega Super Bowl

Servings: 2
Total Time: 25 minutes

Ingredients:
- 1 tablespoon ghee
- 1 shallot, sliced
- 1 garlic clove, minced
- ½ head of broccoli, cut into small florets
- 6 ounces salmon fillet
- ½ cup almond milk
- ½ cup quinoa, cooked
- 1 cup spinach
- 1 teaspoon Himalayan salt
- 1 teaspoon black pepper, crushed
- 2 teaspoons red chili flakes
- 2 teaspoons flaxseeds oil

Directions:
1. In a medium skillet over medium heat, add ghee, shallot and garlic. Cook 2 minutes and then add the broccoli. Let sauté 8 minutes until broccoli is softened. Remove broccoli and set aside.
2. Place salmon in the same skillet and add almond milk. Bring to a boil, cover the pan and reduce heat. Let simmer for 7 minutes or until fish is cooked through.
3. Set aside salmon and add back to the pan the broccoli, and also add quinoa and spinach. Cook for 3 minutes then season with the salt and pepper. Transfer to serving bowls.
4. Gently flake the salmon and divide among the bowls. Sprinkle with chili flakes, drizzle with flaxseeds oil and serve.

314 - Mediterranean Mushrooms

Servings: 2
Total Time: 20 minutes

Ingredients:
- 4 Portobello mushrooms, stems removed.
- 2 tablespoons olive oil
- 1 zucchini diced
- ¼ cup sun dried tomatoes, chopped
- ¼ cup of sun ripened black olives
- 1 ½ cups quinoa, cooked
- 1 handful of parsley leaves, finely chopped
- 1 handful of cilantro, finely chopped
- 1 tablespoon of pine nuts
- 1 tablespoon of lemon juice
- 1 teaspoon dried oregano
- 1 teaspoon Himalayan salt
- 1 teaspoon black pepper, crushed

Directions:
1. Line a baking tray with parchment paper and place mushrooms stems side up. Drizzle with 1 tablespoon olive oil and gently massage into the mushroom. Place under the broiler on high heat and cook 4 minutes and then flip and cook 4 more minutes.
2. Add 1 tablespoon olive oil to a medium skillet over medium heat along with the zucchini, tomatoes and olives. Cook 5 minutes and then add the quinoa and cook for another 3 minutes. Turn heat off and stir in the parsley, cilantro, pine nuts, lemon juice, oregano, salt and pepper.
3. Top each mushroom with the vegetable and quinoa mixture and serve warm.

315 - Cauliflower Lettuce Cups

Servings: 2
Total Time: 20 minutes

Ingredients:
- ½ cauliflower head, chopped into small pieces
- 1 tablespoon coconut oil
- 1 carrot, grated
- 1 cup mushrooms, diced
- 2 shallots, diced
- 1 garlic clove, finely diced
- 1 inch piece of ginger, grated
- 1 tablespoon coconut aminos
- 1 tablespoon tamari
- 1 lime, juiced
- 1 teaspoon Himalayan salt
- 1 teaspoon red chili flakes
- 6 large romaine lettuce leaves
- 1 tablespoon cilantro, chopped
- 1 tablespoon walnuts, chopped

Directions:
1. Add cauliflower pieces to a food processor and pulse a few times until it forms a rice-like consistency.
2. Place coconut oil in a medium skillet and heat over medium heat. Add carrot, mushrooms, shallot, garlic and ginger to cook for 8 minutes.
3. Toss in cauliflower, coconut aminos, tamari, lime juice, salt and chili flakes. Cook another 5 minutes until vegetables are tender.
4. Spoon mixture into each lettuce leaf and garnish with cilantro and walnuts before serving.

316 - Citrus Stir Fry

Servings: 2
Total Time: 10 minutes

Ingredients:
- 1 teaspoon sesame oil
- 1 teaspoon coconut oil
- 1 shallot, sliced
- 1 garlic clove, crushed
- ½ cup carrot, shredded
- ½ red bell pepper, seeds removed and sliced
- 1 cup of bok choy, roughly chopped
- 1 tablespoon lime zest
- 1 lime, juiced
- 1 tablespoon fresh ginger, grated
- 3 tablespoons coconut aminos
- 3 tablespoons tamari
- 2 tablespoons water
- 1 zucchini, spiralized into zoodles
- 2 tablespoons cashews
- 2 tablespoons green onions, sliced
- 2 tablespoons cilantro, chopped

Directions:
1. Heat oils in a medium skillet or wok over medium-high heat. Add shallot, garlic, carrot, bell pepper and bok choy. Cook for 3 minutes, stirring frequently.
2. Add lime zest, lime juice, ginger, coconut aminos, tamari and water. Cook another 1 minute and turn off heat.
3. Toss in zoodles and transfer to a serving bowl.
4. Garnish with cashews, green onions and cilantro.

317 - Pineapple Boats

Servings: 2
Total Time: 25 minutes

Ingredients:
- 1 teaspoon coconut oil
- 1 baby bok choy, sliced
- 1 large carrot, diced
- 1 red bell pepper, diced
- 1 garlic clove, minced
- 1 inch piece ginger, grated
- ½ teaspoon turmeric
- 1 teaspoon red chili flakes
- ½ teaspoon cayenne
- ½ cup coconut cream
- 1 cup water
- 1 pineapple, halved lengthwise and flesh taken (to form a boat with the skin), flesh diced
- 1 cup kale, stems removed and chopped
- ½ cup raw cashews, crushed
- 1 cup quinoa, cooked
- 1 tablespoon cilantro, chopped

Directions:
1. Add coconut oil to a large skillet over medium-high heat. Add bok choy, carrot, bell pepper, garlic and ginger and cook for 6 minutes.
2. Stir in turmeric, chili flakes, cayenne, coconut cream, water and diced pineapple. Reduce heat to medium-low and simmer 8 minutes.
3. Add kale, cashews and quinoa to the skillet and cook 2 minutes.
4. Place vegetable and quinoa mixture in the pineapple skin and garnish with cilantro.

---

318 - Moroccan Vegetable Stew

Servings: 2
Total Time: 55 minutes

Ingredients:
- 1 tablespoon olive oil
- ½ cup red onion, chopped
- 1 garlic clove, minced
- 1 carrot, chopped
- 1 sweet potatoes, chopped
- ½ teaspoon coriander
- ½ teaspoon cardamom
- ¼ teaspoon turmeric
- 1 tablespoon fresh ginger root, minced
- 1 large eggplant, chopped
- ½ cup cauliflower, chopped
- ¾ cup vegetable stock
- 1 ½ tablespoon tomato paste
- 1 tablespoon parsley, chopped
- 2 tablespoons mint, chopped
- 1 teaspoon Himalayan salt
- ¼ teaspoon black pepper
- 1 tablespoon lemon zest
- 6-8 green olives

Directions:
1. In a large stockpot add the olive oil, red onion, garlic and carrots over medium heat. Cook for 5 minutes and then add the sweet potatoes, coriander, cardamom, turmeric and ginger root. Toss well to coat and cook another 2 minutes.
2. Add vegetable stock and tomato paste. Bring to a boil and then reduce heat to low and simmer with the lid on for 40 minutes.
3. Stir in eggplant, cauliflower, parsley, 1 tablespoon mint, salt, pepper, lemon zest and green olives. Cook an additional 3 minutes and then transfer to serving bowls.
4. Garnish with remaining tablespoon mint.

319 - Quinoa Stuffed Peppers

Servings: 2
Total Time: 25 minutes

Ingredients:
- 2 bell peppers, halved and seeded
- Pinch of Himalayan salt
- 1 teaspoon olive oil
- 1 onion, diced
- 1 garlic clove, minced
- 1 zucchini, diced
- 3 mushrooms, diced
- 1 tomato, diced
- 1 tablespoon dried oregano
- ½ teaspoon dried basil
- ½ teaspoon red chili flakes
- 1 cup quinoa, cooked
- ½ cup fresh parsley, chopped

Directions:
1. Place bell peppers on a baking tray, cut side down, and sprinkle with salt. Place sheet under the broiler on high for 8 minutes or until browned. Flip and cook another 5 minutes.
2. Heat olive oil in a medium skillet over medium-low heat. Add onion, garlic, zucchini and mushrooms. Cook 5 minutes and then add tomato, oregano, basil and chili flakes. Cook for an additional 5 minutes.
3. Stir in quinoa and parsley and remove from heat.
4. Stuff each half of pepper with the quinoa vegetable mixture and place back in the broiler on a baking tray for 6-8 minutes.
5. Serve and enjoy!

320 - Everything Sweet Potato Pizza

Servings: 2
Total Time: 1 hour 15 minutes

Ingredients:
- 2 large sweet potatoes
- 1 garlic clove, minced
- 1 ½ tablespoons coconut oil, melted
- 1 tablespoon chia seeds
- 3 tablespoons water
- 1 ¼ cups gluten free oat flour
- ½ cup almond flour
- 1 tablespoon apple cider vinegar
- 1 teaspoon Himalayan salt
- 1 cup cherry tomatoes, halved
- 1 tablespoon sun dried tomatoes, chopped
- ½ cup black olives, sliced
- 2 tablespoons green onions
- 1 tablespoon nutritional yeast

Spinach Pesto

- 3 cups spinach
- 1 cup basil
- 3 tablespoons olive oil
- 2 garlic cloves
- 1 teaspoon pine nuts
- 1 teaspoon nutritional yeast
- 1 teaspoon Himalayan salt

Directions:
1. Poke holes in the sweet potatoes with a fork and place on a baking tray. Coat with garlic and ½ tablespoon coconut oil.
2. Roast in an oven that has been preheated to 400°F/205°C for 40 minutes or until sweet potatoes are tender. Remove from oven and scoop flesh out of each sweet potato and place in a bowl.
3. Whisk together the chia and water in a small bowl and set aside for 10 minutes
4. Add oat flour, almond flour, remaining coconut oil, vinegar and salt to the sweet potato mixture and stir to combine. Whisk in chia mixture and combine well.
5. On a baking tray lined with parchment paper, form sweet potato dough into a pizza shape. Place in oven and bake for 30 minutes.
6. While pizza cooks, add spinach, basil, olive oil, pine nuts, garlic, salt and nutritional yeast to a food processor or blender. Mix until smooth, adding some more olive oil if necessary to thin out the Spinach Pesto.
7. Once pizza crust is cooked, spread Spinach Pesto on the crust. Top with cherry tomatoes, sun dried tomatoes, olives and green onions. Sprinkle with nutritional yeast and serve.

321 - Lentil Sweet Potato Tacos

Servings: 2
Total Time: 50 minutes

Ingredients:
- 2 medium sweet potatoes
- 1 teaspoon avocado oil
- 1 shallot, sliced
- 1 cup lentils, cooked
- 1 teaspoon cumin
- 1 teaspoon chili powder
- ¼ cup green onion, chopped
- 1 teaspoon lime juice
- 1 teaspoon Himalayan salt
- ¼ cup tomatoes, chopped
- 1 avocado, sliced
- 2 teaspoons unsweetened yogurt
- 1 tablespoon cilantro, chopped

Directions:
1. Poke sweet potatoes with a fork several times and roast in the oven at 400°F/205°C for 40 minutes.
2. While sweet potato cooks, heat oil in a small skillet over medium heat and add shallot, lentils, cumin and chili powder. Cook 5 minutes and then add green onion, lime juice and salt.
3. When sweet potatoes are cooked, make a 2 inch slit in the top of each and open them up. Spoon lentil mixture into each sweet potato and top with tomatoes, avocado, yogurt and cilantro.

322 - Spaghetti Squash and Meatless Meatballs

Servings: 2
Total Time: 1 hour 5 minutes

Ingredients:
- 1 teaspoon olive oil
- 1 spaghetti squash, halved lengthwise and seeds removed
- 1 tablespoon ground flaxseeds
- 3 tablespoons water
- 1 tablespoon coconut oil
- 1 garlic clove, minced
- ½ yellow onion, diced
- ½ cup spinach, chopped
- 1 teaspoon apple cider vinegar
- 1 tablespoon fresh thyme, chopped
- 1 tablespoon fresh parsley, chopped
- 1 teaspoon dried oregano
- 1 teaspoon Himalayan salt
- 1 teaspoon black pepper, crushed
- ½ cup lentils, cooked
- 4 ounces baby bella mushrooms, diced
- ¼ cup quinoa, cooked
- 1 tablespoon almond meal
- ½ cup diced tomatoes

Directions:
1. Preheat oven to 400°F/205°C. Rub olive oil on the flesh side of the squash and on a baking tray lined with parchment paper, place squash cut side down. Roast for 30 minutes or until flesh is tender.
2. In a small bowl, whisk together the flaxseeds with 3 tablespoons water. Set aside.
3. Heat coconut oil in a small skillet over medium heat and add garlic and onions. Cook 5 minutes and then add spinach, sautéing another 2 minutes. Add vinegar, thyme, parsley, oregano, salt and pepper. Remove from heat
4. In a food processor, blend lentils and mushrooms until combined. Transfer to a medium bowl and add quinoa, almond meal as well as the mixture from the small skillet and flax mixture. Combine with your hands until you can form balls. Form dough into balls and place on a baking tray. Bake in oven for 30 minutes.
5. With a fork, remove the flesh from the skin of the squash. Toss in diced tomatoes. Place back in the oven for 10 minutes or until warmed.
6. Top with lentil mushroom balls and serve.

323 - Raw Thai Wraps

Servings: 2
Total Time: 10 minutes

Ingredients:
- ½ zucchini, spiralized into thin noodles
- 1 carrot, shredded
- ½ cup red onion, thinly sliced
- ½ cup scallion, sliced
- ½ bunch kale, stems removed and thinly sliced
- ¼ cup red cabbage, shredded
- 2 tablespoons sesame seeds
- 1 teaspoon Himalayan salt
- 1 teaspoon avocado oil
- 1 teaspoon lemon juice
- 3-4 big romaine leaves

Peanut Sauce
- 1 tablespoon of sesame oil
- 1 tablespoon apple cider vinegar
- 2 tablespoons natural peanut butter
- 1 teaspoon coconut aminos
- 1 teaspoon lime juice
- 1 teaspoon cilantro, chopped

Directions:
1. In a medium sized bowl, combine zucchini noodles, carrot, red onion, scallion, kale, cabbage, sesame seeds, salt, avocado oil and lemon juice. Toss well and let sit for 5 minutes in the fridge.
2. Make the Peanut Sauce by whisking together the sesame oil, vinegar, peanut butter, coconut aminos, lime juice and cilantro in a small bowl.
3. Place romaine leaves on a platter and spoon the vegetable mixture evenly into each one.
4. Drizzle sauce over each wrap and serve immediately.

324 - Eggplant & Chickpea Stew

Servings: 2
Total Time: 30 minutes

Ingredients:
- 1 large eggplant, halved
- 1 teaspoon olive oil, divided
- 1 cup yellow onion, finely diced
- 2 cups tomatoes, diced
- ½ teaspoon fresh ginger, grated
- ½ teaspoon fresh garlic, grated
- ½ teaspoon coriander powder
- 1 teaspoon cumin powder
- ⅛ teaspoon turmeric
- ¼ teaspoon cinnamon
- ½ teaspoon red chili flakes
- 2 tablespoons water
- ¼ teaspoon Himalayan salt
- 1 cup chickpeas, cooked
- 2 tablespoons cilantro, chopped

Directions:
1. Preheat oven to 375°F/190°C. Line a baking tray with parchment paper.
2. Place eggplant, cut side down, on the baking tray and roast for 20 minutes.
3. In a large skillet heat olive oil over medium-low heat. Add onion and cook for 5 minutes. Stir in the tomatoes, ginger, garlic, coriander, cumin, turmeric, cinnamon, chili flakes water and salt. Cook for another 5 minutes before adding the chickpeas.
4. Remove eggplant from the oven, remove the skin and chop into pieces. Toss eggplant into the large skillet with the tomato, spice and chickpea mixture.
5. Cook for 2 minutes and then transfer to serving bowl and garnish with cilantro.

325 - Mushroom, Onion & Brown Rice Sauté

Servings: 2
Total Time: 15 minutes

Ingredients:
- 2 tablespoons olive oil, divided
- 2 shallots, thinly sliced
- 2 garlic cloves, minced
- 1 teaspoon ginger, grated
- ¼ teaspoon red chili flakes
- ½ pound crimini mushrooms, sliced
- ½ teaspoon Himalayan salt
- ½ teaspoon black pepper. Crushed
- 1 cup brown rice, cooked
- 1 tablespoon apple cider vinegar
- 1 tablespoon tamari
- 1 tablespoon coconut aminos
- ½ cup arugula
- 1 tablespoon pine nuts, toasted

Directions:
1. Heat oil in a medium skillet over medium heat and add shallots, garlic, ginger and red chili flakes. Cook 3 minutes and then add mushrooms, salt and black pepper.
2. Cook 8 minutes and then add the rice, vinegar, tamari and coconut aminos. Cook for 2 minutes.
3. Place arugula in a large bowl and top with mushroom and rice mixture. Garnish with pine nuts and serve immediately.

326 - Tofu Ginger Stir-Fry

Servings: 2
Total Time: 25 minutes

Ingredients:
- 1 tablespoon sesame oil, divided
- 8 ounces firm tofu, cubed
- 1 garlic clove, minced
- 2 shallots, diced
- 2 tablespoons green onion, sliced
- 1-inch piece ginger, minced
- ¼ teaspoon turmeric
- ½ teaspoon red chili flakes
- 1 tablespoon tamari
- 2 cups Napa cabbage, shredded
- ½ cup fresh shiitake mushrooms
- 1 cup broccoli, cut into florets
- ¼ cup edamame
- 1 zucchini, spiralized into thin noodles
- 1 tablespoon sesame seeds
- 1 tablespoon cilantro, chopped

Directions:
1. Heat half of the oil in a large skillet over medium-high heat. Place tofu and sear on all sides of the cube for a minute each side. Remove tofu from the pan.
2. Add remaining oil and the garlic, shallot, green onion, ginger, turmeric, red chili flakes and tamari. Cook for 2 minutes, stirring frequently. Add cabbage, mushrooms, broccoli and edamame.
3. Cook 8-10 minutes or until vegetables are soft. Toss in zucchini noodles and tofu and cook an additional 2 minutes.
4. Transfer to serving bowl and top with sesame seeds and cilantro.

327 - Cashew Vegetable Skillet

Servings: 2
Total Time: 15 minutes

Ingredients:
- 1 tablespoon coconut oil
- ½ red onion, thinly sliced
- 2 garlic cloves, minced
- 1 celery stalk, sliced
- ½ red bell pepper, sliced
- 1 small green chili, seeds removed and diced
- ½ cup raw cashews, toasted
- ½ cup broccoli, cut into florets
- ½ cup cauliflower, cut into florets
- 10 snow pea pods
- 2 tablespoons green onions, sliced
- 1 tablespoon sesame seeds
- 1 tablespoon cilantro, chopped

Sauce
- 1 cup vegetable broth
- 3 tablespoons coconut aminos
- 1 tablespoon tamari
- 1 tablespoon raw honey
- 1 tablespoon sesame oil
- 2 teaspoons apple cider vinegar
- ½ teaspoon red chili flakes
- ½ teaspoon ground ginger
- ⅛ teaspoon ground cloves
- ⅛ teaspoon black pepper, crushed
- 2 teaspoons cornstarch

Directions:
1. Make the Sauce by whisking the Sauce ingredients together in a medium bowl until well combined.
2. In a large skillet, heat oil over medium-high heat and sauté the onion, garlic, celery, pepper and chili. After 5 minutes add the cashews, broccoli and cauliflower. Cook 2 minutes and then add the Sauce.
3. Continue cooking for 3 minutes and then add the snow peas. Cook 1 minute.
4. Transfer to serving bowl and garnish with green onion, sesame seeds and cilantro.

328 - Fried Broccoli Rice

Servings: 2
Total Time: 20 minutes

Ingredients:
- 1 tablespoon coconut oil
- 2 shallots, sliced
- 1 small head broccoli, cut into florets
- ½ cup brown rice, cooked and cooled
- 1/3 cup cashews, toasted
- 1 tablespoon green onion, sliced

Sauce
- 2 tablespoons tamari
- 1 tablespoon water
- 1 teaspoon coconut aminos
- 1 teaspoon raw honey
- 1 teaspoon sesame oil
- 1 teaspoon rice wine vinegar
- 1 teaspoon lime juice
- ½ teaspoon red chili flakes
- ½ teaspoon ginger, grated
- 1 garlic clove, minced
- ⅛ teaspoon cloves

Directions:
1. Make the Sauce by whisking the Sauce ingredients together in a medium bowl until well combined.
2. In a large skillet, heat oil over medium-high heat and sauté the shallot. Cook 5 minutes and then add the broccoli.
3. Continue cooking for 5 minutes and then add the rice and sauce, making sure to stir well.
4. Cook 5 minutes and then transfer to serving bowl and garnish with cashews and green onion.

329 - Coconut Lentil Stew

Servings: 2
Total Time: 35 minutes

Ingredients:
- 1 tablespoon coconut oil
- ½ teaspoon cumin seeds
- ¼ teaspoon mustard seeds
- ¼ teaspoon fenugreek seeds
- 2 shallots, sliced
- 1-inch piece ginger, grated
- ¼ teaspoon cayenne
- ½ teaspoon ground coriander
- ½ teaspoon ground cumin
- ¼ teaspoon turmeric
- ¼ teaspoon cinnamon
- ½ teaspoon Himalayan salt
- ½ teaspoon black pepper, crushed
- ¾ cup split red lentils
- 1 tomato, diced
- 1 ½ cups water
- ¼ cup coconut milk
- ½ lime, juiced
- 3 cups kale, stems removed and thinly sliced
- 2 tablespoons coconut flakes, toasted
- 2 tablespoons cilantro

Directions:
1. Heat half of the oil in a medium saucepan over medium heat and add the cumin seeds, mustard seeds, fenugreek seeds and shallots. Cook 5 minutes until shallots are soft and spices are fragrant. Add ginger and cook another minute before adding the cayenne, coriander, cumin, turmeric and cinnamon.
2. Cook spices for 2 minutes and then add the salt, pepper, lentils, tomato and water. Bring to a boil and then reduce heat to low and simmer 10 minutes. Add the coconut milk and lime juice and continue cooking for 10 more minutes.
3. In a small saucepan, heat remaining coconut oil and quickly sauté the kale, about 5 minutes or until it has wilted.
4. Transfer mixture from the medium saucepan to a bowl, top with sautéed kale, coconut flakes and cilantro. Serve warm.

330 - Noodle & Pesto Pizza

Servings: 2
Total Time: 30 minutes

Ingredients:
- 1 medium sweet potato, spiralized into thin noodles
- 1 tablespoon almond meal
- 1 tablespoon flaxseeds meal
- 1 tablespoon coconut oil
- ¼ teaspoon cumin powder

Pesto

- ½ cup kale
- 1 garlic clove
- 1 tablespoon olive oil
- 1 lemon, juiced
- 1 ½ tablespoons pine nuts
- ¼ teaspoon Himalayan salt
- ¼ teaspoon black pepper, crushed

Topping

- 1 ½ tablespoon olive oil
- 1 ½ cups arugula
- 1 teaspoon lemon juice
- ½ teaspoon oregano
- ¼ teaspoon Himalayan salt
- 1 small tomato, sliced
- ½ small avocado, sliced

Directions:
1. Preheat oven to 425°F/220°C.
2. Mix sweet potato, almond meal, flaxseeds meal, coconut oil and cumin together in a medium bowl. Heat a medium, oven-safe skillet over high heat and add the sweet potato mixture, ensuring that it is in a circular shape and pressed down evenly. Cook 5 minutes.
3. Transfer skillet to the oven and cook for 10 minutes.
4. Make the Pesto by adding all the Pesto ingredients to a blender and processing until smooth. Set aside.
5. After 10 minutes, flip sweet potato crust onto a baking tray lined with parchment paper so that the side that had been down in the pan now faces up. Drizzle with the ½ tablespoon of olive oil and place back in the oven for another 10 minutes.
6. In a small bowl, place the arugula, 1 tablespoon olive oil, lemon juice, oregano and salt. Toss well to coat.
7. Remove sweet potato crust and spread pesto on top. Arrange tomato and avocado slices in alternating pattern and then top with arugula.

331 - Farmer's Market Salad

Servings: 2
Total Time: 10 minutes

Ingredients:
- 1 cup quinoa, cooked
- 2 garlic cloves, minced
- ½ red onion, diced
- ½ bunch kale, stems removed and cut into thin ribbons
- ½ 15 oz. can of white beans, drained and rinsed
- 1 zucchini, grated
- 1 yellow squash, grated
- 1 tomato, diced
- 1/3 cup fresh basil, sliced into ribbons
- 2 tablespoons pumpkin seeds
- 1 lemon, zested and juiced
- 2 tablespoons olive oil
- ½ teaspoon Himalayan salt
- ½ teaspoon black pepper, crushed
- 1 tablespoon parsley, chopped

Directions:
1. In a large bowl, combine all ingredients (except for parsley) and toss well to coat. Let sit 5 minutes so kale softens.
2. Garnish with parsley before serving.

332 - Kale Chard Warm Salad

Servings: 2
Total Time: 10 minutes

Ingredients:
- 2 tablespoons olive oil
- 1 bunch of kale, stems removed and thinly sliced
- 1 bunch of rainbow chard, stems removed and thinly sliced
- 1 cup red cabbage, thinly shredded
- ½ cup sauerkraut
- 1 garlic clove, minced
- ½ lemon, zested and juiced
- ½ teaspoon apple cider vinegar
- ¼ teaspoon Himalayan salt
- ½ teaspoon black pepper, crushed
- 1 cup brown rice, cooked
- 1 tablespoon parsley

Directions:
1. Heat olive oil in a medium skillet over medium-low heat. Add kale, chard, and cabbage and cook 5-7 minutes or until wilted.
2. Add in sauerkraut, garlic, lemon zest and juice, vinegar, salt and pepper. Cook 1 additional minute.
3. Serve on top of warm brown rice and garnish with parsley.

333 - Veggie Medley Skillet

Servings: 2
Total Time: 35 minutes

Ingredients:
- 1 small sweet potato
- 3 small eggplants, diced
- 1 cup zucchini, sliced
- 1 teaspoon coconut oil
- 2 garlic cloves, minced
- ½-inch piece ginger, minced
- 2 cups arugula leaves
- 1 lemon, juiced
- 1 teaspoon maple syrup
- ½ teaspoon cayenne pepper
- 1 tomato, diced
- 1 cucumber, sliced
- 1 tablespoon walnuts, crushed
- ½ teaspoon Himalayan salt
- ½ teaspoon black pepper, crushed

Directions:
1. Preheat oven to 350°F/180°C. Poke holes in sweet potato with a fork and rub the eggplant and zucchini with coconut oil. Arrange in sections in a large oven-safe skillet (such as a cast iron pan). Sprinkle with garlic and ginger.
2. Roast in the oven for 30 minutes or until vegetables are soft.
3. While vegetables are roasting, combine the arugula, lemon juice, maple syrup, cayenne, tomato, cucumber, walnuts, salt and pepper in a large bowl and toss well to coat.
4. After 30 minutes, remove skillet from the oven and top with arugula mixture.
5. Serve from the skillet.

334 - Indian Onion & Peppers

Servings: 2
Total Time: 20 minutes

Ingredients:
- 1 ½ tablespoons coconut oil
- 1 medium yellow onion, chopped
- 1 small shallot, sliced
- ½ green bell pepper, chopped
- ½ red bell pepper, chopped
- 2 garlic cloves, chopped
- 1 green chili, chopped
- 1-inch piece ginger, grated
- 1 teaspoon cumin seeds
- ½ teaspoon turmeric powder
- 1 tablespoon cashews
- 3 tablespoons tomato paste
- ½ cup diced tomatoes
- ½ teaspoon garam masala powder
- 1 teaspoon red chili powder
- ½ teaspoon cayenne pepper
- ½ teaspoon Himalayan salt
- 1 tablespoon cilantro, chopped

Directions:
1. Heat coconut oil in a medium pot over medium-high heat. Add the onion, shallot, bell peppers, garlic, chili and ginger. Cook for 8 minutes, stirring occasionally, and then add the cumin seeds, turmeric and cashews.
2. Cook another 3 minutes before adding the tomato paste, diced tomatoes, garam masala, chili powder, cayenne pepper and salt.
3. Cook 5 more minutes and remove from heat.
4. Garnish with cilantro and serve.

---

335 - Broccoli Pasta

Servings: 2
Total Time: 30 minutes

Ingredients:
- 1 small head of broccoli, cut into florets
- 1 ½ tablespoons coconut oil
- 1 garlic clove, minced
- 1 zucchini, spiralized into noodles
- ½ teaspoon red pepper flakes
- ½ yellow onion, thinly sliced
- 1 tablespoon parsley, chopped
- 1 cup lentils, cooked
- ½ teaspoon Himalayan salt
- ½ teaspoon black pepper, crushed
- 1 tablespoon nutritional yeast

Directions:
1. Preheat oven to 400°F/205°C. Line a baking tray with parchment paper. In a medium bowl, toss broccoli with the ½ tablespoon coconut oil and garlic. Place in an even layer on the baking tray.
2. Roast broccoli in the oven for 25 minutes or until tender.
3. Heat remaining oil in a medium skillet over medium heat. Add zucchini, red pepper flakes, onion and parsley. Cook 5 minutes then add the lentils, salt, pepper and broccoli mixture from the oven. Continuously stir for 1 minute.
4. Garnish with nutritional yeast and serve warm.

336 - Roasted Vegetable, Hummus & Quinoa Bake

Servings: 2
Total Time: 40 minutes

Ingredients:
- 1 cup fresh tomatoes, diced
- 3 shallots, sliced
- 2 small zucchinis, cubed
- 1 cup broccoli, florets cut into small pieces
- 1 yellow bell pepper, chopped
- 2 garlic cloves, minced
- 2 tablespoons coconut oil
- ½ teaspoon Himalayan salt
- ½ teaspoon black pepper, crushed
- ½ teaspoon turmeric
- 1 tablespoon parsley
- 1 cup quinoa, cooked
- 1 ½ cups hummus
- 2 tablespoons nutritional yeast

Directions:
1. Preheat oven to 400°F/205°C. Line a baking tray with parchment paper. In a medium bowl, toss tomatoes, shallots, zucchini, broccoli, bell pepper and garlic with 1 ½ tablespoons coconut oil, salt, pepper and turmeric. Place on the baking tray in an even layer and roast in the oven for 25 minutes or until tender.
2. In a small bowl, combine the parsley and quinoa.
3. Grease a small glass baking dish with the remaining ½ tablespoon coconut oil. Place quinoa in a single layer on the bottom of the dish. Spread a layer of hummus on top of the quinoa. Top with roasted vegetables.
4. Sprinkle with nutritional yeast and bake in the oven for 10 minutes.
5. Remove and serve immediately.

337 - Spicy Pepper Soup

Servings: 2
Total Time: 55 minutes

Ingredients:
- 1 yellow squash, diced
- ¼ red bell pepper, chopped
- 1 shallot, sliced
- 1 tablespoon coconut oil
- ½ 15 ounce can coconut milk
- 2 teaspoons red curry paste
- ½ teaspoon turmeric powder
- 1 lime, juiced
- ½ teaspoon Himalayan salt
- 1 cup brown rice, cooked
- 1 tablespoon cilantro, chopped
- 1 tablespoon cashews, toasted

Directions:
1. Preheat oven to 375°F/190°C. Line a baking tray with parchment paper. Toss squash, bell pepper and shallot with coconut oil in a medium bowl. Place on the baking tray in an even layer. Roast in the oven for 30 minutes or until tender.
2. In a medium saucepan, heat coconut milk, curry paste and turmeric over medium heat until red curry paste is completely dissolved, about 8 minutes.
3. Remove vegetables from the oven and let cool for 5 minutes. Then, add to a food processor along with the coconut milk/curry mixture, lime juice and salt. Blend until smooth.
4. Return to the medium saucepan and bring to a boil. Reduce heat to low and simmer 10 minutes.
5. Serve along with brown rice and garnish with cilantro and cashews.

338 - Rainbow Spaghetti Squash

Servings: 2
Total Time: 30 minutes

Ingredients:
- 2 tablespoons coconut oil, divided
- 1 spaghetti squash, halved lengthwise and seeds removed
- ½ red onion, thinly sliced
- 1 orange bell pepper, sliced
- 1 cup red cabbage, thinly sliced
- 2 green onions, sliced
- 1 cup kale, stems removed and thinly sliced
- 1 cup quinoa, quinoa
- 2 teaspoon dried thyme
- 1 teaspoon oregano
- 1 teaspoon garlic powder
- ½ teaspoon Himalayan salt
- ½ teaspoon black pepper, crushed
- 1 tablespoon pine nuts, toasted
- 1 tablespoon parsley, chopped
- 1 tablespoon nutritional yeast

Directions:
1. Preheat oven to 400°F/205°C. Line a baking tray with parchment paper. Brush 1 tablespoon of oil on the cut sides of the squash and place cut side down on the baking tray.
2. Roast in the oven for 25 minutes or until tender.
3. While squash cooks, add remaining oil to a medium saucepan and add onion, bell pepper, cabbage and green onions. Cook 8 minutes until vegetables are softened. Stir in kale and cook another 3 minutes. Add quinoa, thyme, oregano, garlic powder, salt and pepper. Cook 2 more minutes and turn off the heat.
4. Remove the squash from the oven and, with a fork, loosen some of the flesh of the squash. Spoon half the quinoa and vegetable mixture into each squash half.
5. Garnish with pine nuts, parsley and nutritional yeast before serving.

---

339 - Sweet Tofu & Vegetables

Servings: 2
Total Time: 25 minutes

Ingredients:
- 1 tablespoon coconut oil
- ½ cup carrot, sliced
- 2 shallots, sliced
- 1 cup red cabbage, thinly shredded
- ½ cup red bell pepper, seeded, and sliced
- 2 cups broccoli, cut into florets
- ¼ teaspoon red chili flakes
- 6 ounces tofu, cubed and baked
- ½ cup cashews, chopped
- 1 tablespoon cilantro, chopped

Sauce

- ½ tablespoon arrowroot powder
- ½ tablespoon roughly chopped fresh ginger
- 2 garlic cloves
- ¼ cup water
- 2 tablespoons tamari
- 1 tablespoon coconut aminos
- 1 tablespoon maple syrup
- ¼ tablespoon lime juice
- 1 tablespoon cilantro

Directions:
1. Prepare the Sauce by adding all the Sauce ingredients to a blender and mixing until smooth. Set aside.
2. Heat coconut oil in a medium skillet over medium-high heat and add carrot, shallot, cabbage, bell pepper and broccoli. Sauté for 10 minutes and then add chili flakes and tofu. Cook another 5 minutes before adding the Sauce.
3. Lower heat to low and let Sauce come to a light simmer. Add cashews and cook for another 2 minutes.
4. Garnish with cilantro before serving.

340 - Lime Green Pasta

Servings: 2
Total Time: 10 minutes

Ingredients:
- 2 zucchinis, spiralized
- 1 cup edamame, shelled and cooked
- 2 tablespoons green onions
- 1 green bell pepper, seeded and thinly sliced
- 1 cup green cabbage, thinly shredded

Lime Sauce
- 1 ripe avocado, pit and skin removed
- ½ cup spinach
- ¼ cup fresh cilantro
- 1 lime, juiced
- ½ cup water
- 1 teaspoon raw honey
- ½ teaspoon tamari
- ¼ teaspoon coconut aminos
- ¼ teaspoon Himalayan salt
- ¼ teaspoon black pepper, crushed
- ¼ teaspoon cayenne

Directions:
1. Prepare the Lime Sauce by adding all the Lime Sauce ingredients to a blender and processing until smooth. Set aside.
2. In a large bowl, combine the zucchini, edamame, green onions, bell pepper and cabbage. Pour Lime Sauce on top and toss until well coated.
3. Serve immediately.

341 - Roasted Eggplant & Quinoa

Servings: 2
Total Time: 30 minutes plus 1 hour of resting

Ingredients:
- 2 small eggplants, cut into cubes
- ¾ teaspoon Himalayan salt
- 1 tablespoon olive oil
- ¼ teaspoon dried thyme
- ¼ teaspoon dried oregano
- 2 tablespoons sesame seeds
- 1 cup quinoa, cooked
- 1 cup arugula
- ¼ cup pine nuts, toasted
- ¼ cup golden raisins
- ¼ teaspoon nutmeg
- ½ cup parsley, chopped
- ¼ cup mint, chopped
- 1 lemon, zested and juiced

Directions:
1. Place eggplant cubes in a colander in the sink or over a bowl. Sprinkle with ½ teaspoon of salt and let sit for 1 hour. Rinse and pat dry.
2. Preheat oven to 400°F/205°C and line a baking tray with parchment paper. In a medium bowl, combine the eggplant, olive oil, thyme, oregano, ¼ teaspoon salt and sesame seeds. Place eggplant on baking tray and roast in the oven for 20 minutes, flipping once halfway through.
3. In a large bowl, combine the roasted eggplant, quinoa, arugula, pine nuts, raisins, nutmeg, parsley, mint and lemon juice.
4. Garnish with lemon zest and serve immediately.

DESSERT RECIPES

342 - Minted Fruit Salad

Servings: 2
Total Time: 20 minutes

Ingredients:
- 2 teaspoons raw honey
- 1 lime, juiced
- 1 tablespoon fresh mint, chopped
- Pinch Himalayan salt
- ½ cup raspberries
- ½ cup blackberries
- 1/3 cup blueberries
- ½ cup pineapple, diced

Directions:
1. In a small bowl mix together the honey, lime juice, mint and pinch of salt.
2. In a large bowl combine the raspberries, blackberries, blueberries and pineapple.
3. Pour the honey mint mixture over the fruit and toss to combine. Let sit for 15 minutes before serving.

343 - Apricot Tarts

Servings: Makes 8 tarts
Total Time: 30 minutes

Ingredients:
- ½ cup raw almonds
- ¾ cup dried dates, pitted and soaked for 15 minutes
- 1 teaspoon nutmeg
- 1 teaspoon cinnamon
- ½ teaspoon Himalayan salt
- 2 small apricots, sliced into 16 pieces
- 8 small mint leaves

Cashew Filling
- ½ cup raw cashews, soaked for 1 hour and drained
- 3 tablespoons lemon juice
- ½ tablespoon lemon zest
- 3 tablespoons water
- 1 teaspoon vanilla extract
- 1 teaspoon raw honey
- ½ teaspoon Himalayan salt

Directions:
1. Make tarts shell dough by combining the almonds, drained dates, nutmeg, cinnamon and salt in a food processor. Pulse until mixture becomes crumbly then continue to blend until a slightly sticky ball forms.
2. Remove tart shell dough from food processor and form into 8 equal sized balls. Press down each ball into a mini muffin or tart pan, making sure to create equal sides. Place pan in fridge for 10 minutes and then remove the shells.
3. In a clean food processor, combine the Cashew Filling ingredients until smooth. Place in a bowl and let chill for 10 minutes.
4. In each tart shell, add the Cashew Filling and top with two apricot slices and a mint leaf.

344 - Sweet Potato Tarts

Servings: Makes 8 tarts
Total Time: 40 minutes

Ingredients:
- ½ cup raw almonds
- ¾ cup dried dates, pitted and soaked for 15 minutes
- 1 teaspoon nutmeg
- 1 teaspoon cinnamon
- ½ teaspoon Himalayan salt

Sweet Potato Filling

- 2 small sweet potatoes, peeled and cut into large cubes
- ¼ cup unsweetened almond milk
- 1 teaspoon nutmeg
- 1 teaspoon cinnamon
- ½ teaspoon vanilla extract

Whipped Coconut Cream (optional)

- 1 can full fat coconut milk, chilled overnight in the fridge
- ½ teaspoon vanilla extract
- ½ teaspoon lemon zest
- 1 tablespoon maple syrup

Directions:
1. Make tarts shell dough by combining the almonds, drained dates, nutmeg, cinnamon and salt in a food processor. Pulse until mixture becomes crumbly then continue to blend until a slightly sticky ball forms.
2. Remove tart shell dough from food processor and form into 8 equal sized balls. Press down each ball into a mini muffin or tart pan, making sure to create equal sides. Place pan in fridge for 10 minutes and then remove the shells.
3. Place sweet potato in a medium saucepan and cover with water. Bring to a boil over medium heat and then reduce heat to low and simmer for 15 minutes or until sweet potatoes are soft.
4. Transfer sweet potatoes to the food processor and add almond milk, nutmeg, cinnamon and vanilla extract. Blend until smooth and chill for 10 minutes.
5. If using the Whipped Coconut Cream, open the can of coconut milk and drain the water for later use. Add coconut cream to a bowl (preferably a chilled metal bowl) and add the vanilla, zest and maple syrup. Beat with a hand mixer for 3 minutes or until fluffy.
6. In each tart shell, add the Sweet Potato Filling and top with the Whipped Coconut Cream. Chill before serving.

---

345 - Creamy Tropical Ice Pops

Servings: Makes 4 popsicles
Total Time: 5 minutes plus 8 hours of freeze time

Ingredients:
- ½ cup pineapple, cubed (not frozen)
- ½ banana
- ½ cup cashews, soaked overnight and drained
- 1 cup unsweetened coconut milk (from can)
- 2 dates, pitted, soaked 15 minutes and drained
- ½ teaspoon vanilla extract
- 1 teaspoon raw honey

Directions:
1. Blend all ingredients in a high speed blender.
2. Pour mixture into 4 ice pop molds. Halfway through freezing, insert popsicle sticks.
3. Freeze for a total of 8 hours.

346 - Nutty Oatmeal Raisin Cookies

Servings: Makes 12 cookies
Total Time: 25 minutes

Ingredients:
- 1 cup spelt flour
- ½ teaspoon baking soda
- ½ teaspoon salt
- 1 cup gluten free rolled oats
- 1/3 cup almond butter, melted
- 2 tablespoons olive oil
- 1 cup coconut sugar
- 1/3 cup unsweetened almond milk
- 1 teaspoon vanilla extract
- ¼ cup raisins
- ¼ cup walnuts
- ½ cup slivered almonds
- 2 tablespoons dried currants

Directions:
1. Preheat oven to 400°F/205°C. Prepare baking tray by lining with parchment paper.
2. In a small bowl, sift together the flour, baking soda and salt. Stir in oats.
3. In a large bowl whisk together the almond butter, olive oil, coconut sugar, almond milk and vanilla extract.
4. Add dry ingredients to the wet ingredients and stir well to combine. Mix in the raisins, walnuts, almonds and currants.
5. Drop spoonfuls of the cookie dough on baking tray. Bake for approximately 8 - 10 minutes or until cookies start to brown. Cool completely before serving.

347 - Raspberry & Chocolate Mousse Jars

Servings: 2
Total Time: 15 minutes

Ingredients:
- 1 large ripe avocado
- 1/3 cup raw cacao powder
- ¼ cup almond milk
- 3 - 4 dates, pitted, soaked for 15 minutes and drained
- 1 teaspoon vanilla extract
- ¾ cup fresh raspberries
- ¼ teaspoon Himalayan salt
- 1 teaspoon maple syrup (optional)
- 2 tablespoon almond slivers, toasted
- 2 small mint leaves

Directions:
1. In a food processor, puree the avocado until smooth. Add in cacao, almond milk, dates, and vanilla extract. Continue to mix until very smooth and well combined.
2. Add ½ raspberries and salt to the avocado mixture and continue to process in the food processor. Taste and if more sweetness is desired, add in maple syrup.
3. Spoon mixture into 2 jars and top each with the rest of the raspberries, almond slivers and a mint leaf. Chill 5 minutes before serving.

348 - Refreshing Fruit & Cilantro Pops

Servings: Makes 4 popsicles
Total Time: 5 minutes plus 8 hours freeze time

Ingredients:
- ½ cup pineapple cubes
- ½ cup mango cubes
- 2 tablespoons cilantro
- 1 tablespoon lime juice
- ½ banana
- 1 tablespoon raw honey
- ¾ cup coconut water

Directions:
1. Blend all ingredients together in a blender until smooth.
2. Pour into ice pop molds and place in freezer. Halfway through insert popsicle sticks.
3. Freeze for a total of 8 hours.

349 - Lemon Pudding & Raspberry Tarts

Servings: Makes 8 tarts
Total Time: 30 minutes

Ingredients:
- ½ cup raw almonds
- ¾ cup dried dates, pitted and soaked for 15 minutes
- 1 teaspoon lemon zest
- ½ teaspoon Himalayan salt
- 8 fresh raspberries
- 8 small mint leaves

Lemon Pudding
- 2 ½ lemons, juiced
- ¾ cup almond milk
- 3 egg yolks
- 3 ½ tablespoons cornstarch
- ¼ teaspoon Himalayan salt
- 1 cup water
- 1/3 cup raw honey

Directions:
1. Make Lemon Pudding by placing a medium saucepan over medium-low heat and whisking in the lemon juice, almond milk and egg yolks. Continue stirring until mixture comes to a boil. Turn heat off.
2. Mix together the cornstarch, salt and water. Stir into lemon and egg mixture then stir in the honey.
3. Make tarts shell dough by combining the almonds, drained dates, lemon zest and salt in a food processor. Pulse until mixture becomes crumbly then continue to blend until a slightly sticky ball forms.
4. Remove tart shell dough from food processor and form into 8 equal sized balls. Press each ball into a mini muffin or tart pan, making sure to create equal sides. Place pan in fridge for 10 minutes and then remove the shells.
5. Spoon Lemon Pudding into each tart shell. Top each with a raspberry and mint leaf.

350 - Coconut Cashew Figs

Servings: Makes 10 figs
Total Time: 10 minutes

Ingredients:
- 10 dried figs, pitted and split in half
- 10 teaspoons cashew butter
- ¼ cup shredded or ground coconut
- ½ teaspoon cinnamon
- ½ teaspoon nutmeg
- ¼ teaspoon Himalayan salt

Directions:
1. Stuff each fig with 1 teaspoon cashew butter and close two sides together as much as possible.
2. On a small plate, combine the coconut, cinnamon, nutmeg and salt. Roll each fig into the coconut mixture and serve.

351 - Raw Berry Crumble

Servings: 2
Total Time: 30 minutes

Ingredients:
- 1/3 cup blueberries
- 1/3 cup blackberries
- 1/3 cup raspberries
- ½ cup mixed berries
- 2 dates, pitted, soaked 15 minutes and drained
- 2 teaspoons lime juice
- ¼ teaspoon Himalayan salt
- ¼ teaspoon vanilla extract
- 1 teaspoon cinnamon
- ¼ teaspoon nutmeg
- ¼ teaspoon Himalayan salt

Whipped Coconut Cream (optional)

- 1 can full fat coconut milk, chilled overnight in the fridge
- ½ teaspoon vanilla extract
- ½ teaspoon lemon zest
- 1 tablespoon maple syrup

Crumble

- ½ cup pecans
- ½ cup walnuts
- ½ cup dates, pitted, soaked 2-4 hours and drained
- ¼ cup dried coconut

Directions:
1. Place the blueberries, blackberries and raspberries (excluding the ½ cup mixed berries) in a food processor with the dates, lime juice, salt and vanilla extract. Blend until combined well.
2. Toss together fruit mixture with remaining ½ cup of mixed berries in a small bowl. Spread mixture on the bottom of a small glass dish.
3. Clean the food processor and add all the Crumble ingredients to the food processor. Pulse to combine and stop when mixture is desired crumbly texture.
4. Crumble nut mixture over the fruit mixture.
5. If using the Whipped Coconut Cream, open the can of coconut milk and drain the water for later use. Add coconut cream to a bowl (preferably a chilled metal bowl) and add the vanilla, lemon zest and maple syrup. Beat with a hand mixer for 3 minutes or until fluffy. Spoon on top of the crumble.

---

352 - Coco-nutty Cookies

Servings: Makes 8 cookies
Total Time: 15 minutes plus 2 hours chilling

Ingredients:
- 1 cup walnuts
- 1 ½ cup almonds
- 1/3 cup dates, pitted, soaked 15 minutes and
- 2 tablespoons raisins, soaked 15 minutes and drained
- ½ teaspoon almond extract
- ¼ teaspoon vanilla extract
- ¼ teaspoon Himalayan salt
- 2 tablespoons water
- ¼ cup unsweetened, shredded coconut

Directions:
1. Combine all ingredients except the shredded coconut in a food processor until combined but not entirely smooth.
2. Roll dough into tablespoon sized balls. Roll each ball in shredded coconut and place on baking tray lined in parchment paper.
3. Press each ball down slightly to form a cookie shape. Allow to chill for at least 2 hours before serving.

353 - Chocolate Coconut Bites

Servings: Makes 12 bites
Total Time: 25 minutes plus 1 hour 30 minutes chill time

Ingredients:
- ¾ cup (+1 extra tablespoon) finely shredded, unsweetened coconut, divided
- ¼ cup dates, pitted
- 1 tablespoon pecan butter
- 1 tablespoon cacao powder
- ¼ teaspoon Himalayan salt
- ¼ teaspoon vanilla
- 2 tablespoons pecans, crushed

Chocolate Coating

- 3 tablespoons cacao powder
- 3 tablespoons cacao butter, melted
- 1 tablespoon maple syrup
- ¼ teaspoon vanilla extract
- ½ teaspoon Himalayan salt
- Pinch Himalayan salt

Directions:
1. In a food processor, combine ½ cup of the shredded coconut, the dates and pecan butter. Combine until smooth. Add in ¼ coconut, cacao powder, salt and vanilla. Process until a ball of dough forms.
2. Remove dough and shape into 6 balls. Place on a baking tray lined with parchment paper and chill 1 hour in the fridge.
3. After 1 hour, prepare chocolate coating by whisking all the Chocolate Coating ingredients together in a small bowl.
4. Remove chocolate coconut balls from the fridge. On a small plate, combine the pecans and 1 tablespoon shredded coconut. Dip each ball into the chocolate mixture, coating half of the ball and then dipping the chocolate coating in the pecan coconut mixture. Place back on the baking tray and chill again at least 30 minutes before serving.

---

354 - Squash Pudding Parfaits

Servings: 2
Total Time: 30 minutes

Ingredients:
- ½ cup cashews, soaked overnight and drained
- ¼ cup pumpkin puree
- ¼ cup butternut squash puree
- ¼ teaspoon ground cinnamon
- ⅛ teaspoon ground nutmeg
- ⅛ teaspoon ground ginger
- ⅛ teaspoon Himalayan salt
- ⅛ teaspoon allspice
- 1 tablespoon maple syrup
- ¼ cup unsweetened almond milk
- 2 teaspoons melted coconut oil

Whipped Coconut Cream

- 1 can full fat coconut milk, chilled overnight in the fridge (Do not use Lite Coconut Milk)
- ½ teaspoon vanilla extract
- ¼ teaspoon cinnamon
- 1 tablespoon maple syrup

Pumpkin Pecan Praline (Optional)

- 2 tablespoons water
- 4 tablespoons coconut sugar
- ½ teaspoon Himalayan salt
- 2 tablespoons pumpkin seeds
- 2 tablespoons pecans, crushed

Directions:
1. In a food processor, combine the cashews and the next 10 ingredients. Combine until smooth and set in fridge.
2. To make the Whipped Coconut Cream, open the can of coconut milk and drain the water for later use. Add coconut milk to a bowl (preferably a chilled metal bowl) and add the vanilla, cinnamon and maple syrup. Beat with a hand mixer for 3 minutes or until fluffy.
3. If using the Pumpkin Pecan Praline, line a baking tray with parchment paper. In a small saucepan over medium-high heat, add water and sugar. Stir to dissolve and let cook about 5 minutes being cautious not to burn. Add salt, pumpkin seeds and pecans, stirring constantly. Pour mixture out onto baking tray. When completely cooled, break into pieces.
4. In small jars, layer the squash pudding, whipped coconut cream and pumpkin pecan praline to serve.

355 - Blueberry Ice Cream

Servings: 2
Total Time: 15 minutes plus 2 hours freezing

Ingredients:
- 1 ¼ cup blueberries
- 2 tablespoons unsweetened almond milk
- ¼ teaspoon vanilla extract
- ⅛ teaspoon Himalayan salt
- 4 frozen bananas, sliced

Directions:
1. In a food processor or blender combine all ingredients until smooth.
2. Scoop into a large bowl and let chill in the freezer for at least 2 hours before serving.

---

356 - Raspberry Cheesecakes

Servings: Makes 8 tarts
Total Time: 30 minutes

Ingredients:
- ½ cup raw almonds
- ¾ cup dates, pitted and soaked for 15 minutes
- 1 teaspoon nutmeg
- 1 teaspoon cinnamon
- ½ teaspoon Himalayan salt
- 8 raspberries

Raspberry Cheesecake Filling

- ½ cup raw cashews, soaked for 1 hour and drained
- 3 tablespoons lemon juice
- ½ tablespoon lemon zest
- 3 tablespoons water
- ½ cup raspberries
- 1 teaspoon vanilla extract
- ¼ teaspoon almond extract
- 1 teaspoon raw honey
- ½ teaspoon Himalayan salt

Directions:
1. Make tarts shell dough by combining the almonds, dates, nutmeg, cinnamon and salt in a food processor. Pulse until mixture becomes crumbly then continue to blend until a slightly sticky ball forms.
2. Remove tart shell dough from food processor and form into 8 equal sized balls. Press each ball into a mini muffin or tart pan, making sure to create equal sides. Place pan in fridge for 10 minutes and then remove the shells.
3. In a clean food processor, combine the Raspberry Cheesecake Filling ingredients until smooth.
4. In each tart shell, add the Raspberry Cheesecake Filling and top with a raspberry.

---

357 - Double Chocolate Mint Tarts

Servings: Makes 8 tarts
Total Time: 30 minutes

Ingredients:
- ½ cup raw almonds
- ¾ cup dates, pitted, soaked and drained for 15 minutes
- 2 tablespoons raw cacao powder
- ½ teaspoon Himalayan salt
- 1 tablespoon cacao nibs
- 8 small mint leaves

Chocolate Mint Filling

- ½ cup raw cashews, soaked for 1 hour and drained
- 3 tablespoons water
- 1 teaspoon vanilla extract
- ¼ teaspoon mint extract
- 1 tablespoon maple syrup
- ½ teaspoon Himalayan salt

Directions:
1. Make tarts shell dough by combining the almonds, drained dates, cacao powder and salt in a food processor. Pulse until mixture becomes crumbly then continue to blend until a slightly sticky ball forms.
2. Remove tart shell dough from food processor and form into 8 equal sized balls. Press each ball into a mini muffin or tart pan, making sure to create equal sides. Place pan in fridge for 10 minutes and then remove the shells.
3. In a clean food processor, combine the Chocolate Mint Filling ingredients until smooth.
4. In each tart shell, add the Chocolate Mint Filling and top with cacao nibs and mint leaves.

358 - Brown Rice Pudding

Servings: 2
Total Time: 25 minutes

Ingredients:
- 1 teaspoon ghee
- 2 tablespoons raisins
- 1 ½ cups brown rice, cooked
- 2 cups unsweetened almond milk
- 1 teaspoon cinnamon
- ½ teaspoon nutmeg
- ¼ teaspoon cloves
- 1 tablespoon maple syrup
- ¼ teaspoon Himalayan salt
- 1 tablespoon unsweetened, shredded coconut

Directions:
1. Heat ghee in a small saucepan over medium-heat. Add raisins, brown rice, almond milk, cinnamon, nutmeg, cloves, maple syrup and salt.
2. Bring to a boil then reduce heat to low and simmer for 15 minutes or until liquid is absorbed.
3. Garnish with coconut and serve.

359 - Baked Apples with Peanut Butter Sauce

Servings: 2
Total Time: 25 minutes

Ingredients:
- 1 apple, cored and sliced into ½ inch slices
- 1 teaspoon coconut oil, melted
- 1 teaspoon cinnamon
- ½ teaspoon nutmeg
- ¼ teaspoon Himalayan salt
- ¼ teaspoon coconut sugar
- 2 tablespoons walnuts, crushed and toasted

Peanut Butter Sauce

- ¾ cup unsweetened yogurt
- 2 tablespoons peanut butter, melted
- ½ teaspoon cinnamon

Directions:
1. Preheat oven to 375°F/190°C. In a glass baking dish, layer the apple slices so they are slightly overlapping. Pour melted coconut oil over the top and sprinkle with cinnamon, nutmeg, salt and coconut sugar.
2. Place baking dish in the oven and cook for 10 - 15 minutes.
3. In a small bowl, mix together yogurt, peanut butter and cinnamon to create the Peanut Butter Sauce.
4. Remove apples from the oven, drizzle the Peanut Butter Sauce on top and then add walnuts.

360 - Fig Bites

Servings: Makes approx. 12 bites
Total Time: 20 minutes plus 2 hours chill time

Ingredients:
- ½ cup dates, pitted
- ¼ cup raisins
- ¼ cup dried cherries
- ¼ cup figs
- ½ cup almond flour
- 1 teaspoon vanilla extract
- ¼ teaspoon Himalayan salt
- ¼ cup unsweetened, shredded coconut

Directions:
1. In a food processor combine dates, raisin, cherries and figs. Once well combined, begin adding the almond flour. Lastly, add vanilla and salt. Continue to process until a ball of dough forms.
2. Place shredded coconut on a plate. Line a baking tray with parchment paper.
3. Roll the dough into balls (about a tablespoon each) and then roll in shredded coconut. Place on baking tray and place in fridge when all balls are formed.
4. Chill at least 2 hours before serving.

361 - Kiwi Lime Squares

Servings: Makes 10 squares
Total Time: 15 minutes plus 5 hours dehydrating time

Ingredients:
- 1 cup raisins
- 1 cup almonds, soaked and drained
- 1 ½ cup dates
- 1/3 cup lime juice
- 1 kiwi, peeled and chopped
- 1 tablespoon lime zest

Directions:
1. Preheat oven to lowest available setting, preferably 100°F/40°C.
2. Combine raisins and almonds in a food processor until a loose dough/crust texture forms. Press dough into a square 9" baking tray lined with parchment paper.
3. Add dates, lime juice, kiwi and lime zest to blender and combine until smooth.
4. Pour fruit mixture on top of crust and spread into even layer.
5. Dehydrate in the oven for 5 hours before serving.

---

362 - Chocolate Dipped Apricots

Servings: Makes 8 apricots
Total Time: 15 minutes plus 30 minutes chill time

Ingredients:
- 2 tablespoons coconut oil, melted
- 1 tablespoon maple syrup
- 2 teaspoons raw cacao powder
- 8 apricot slices
- 1 tablespoon flaked sea salt

Directions:
1. Line a baking tray with parchment paper.
2. In a small bowl, whisk together the coconut oil, maple syrup and cacao powder. Dip apricot slice halfway into the chocolate mixture.
3. Sprinkle sea salt on chocolate end of the apricot and place on baking tray.
4. Repeat with remaining 7 apricot slices and place tray in the fridge to chill for 30 minutes.

---

363 - Fruit Skewers

Servings: Makes 4 skewers
Total Time: 10 minutes plus 30 minutes chill time

Ingredients:
- 8 raspberries
- 8 pineapple cubes (about ½ inch)
- 8 blueberries
- 8 mango cubes (about ½ inch)
- 8 small mint leaves
- 8 bamboo skewers

Chocolate Sauce

- 2 tablespoons coconut oil, melted
- 1 tablespoon maple syrup
- 2 teaspoons raw cacao powder

Directions:
1. Place fruit and mint on the skewers in the desired pattern.
2. Make chocolate sauce by whisking together the coconut oil, maple syrup and cacao powder until smooth.
3. On a baking tray lined with parchment paper, place fruit skewers.
4. Drizzle with chocolate sauce and chill 30 minutes in the fridge.

364 - Mint Chocolate Mousse

Servings: 2
Total Time: 5 minutes plus 2 hours chilling

Ingredients:
- 1 10 ounce package silken tofu
- 2 teaspoons raw cacao powder
- ½ teaspoon vanilla extract
- ½ teaspoon peppermint extract
- ¼ teaspoon Himalayan salt
- 1 teaspoon raw honey
- 1 tablespoon cacao nibs
- 4 small mint leaves

Directions:
1. In a food processor, blend together all ingredients except the cacao nibs and mint leaves until smooth.
2. Pour into two cups and chill in the fridge for 2 hours or until ready to serve. Garnish with cacao nibs and mint leaves before serving.

365 - Raw Chocolate Donut Holes

Servings: 2
Total Time: 10 minutes plus 2 hours chilling

Ingredients:
- ½ cup raw walnuts
- ½ cup raw almonds
- 10 dates, pitted and soaked 15 minutes then drained
- ½ tablespoon coconut oil
- ⅛ teaspoon Himalayan pink sea salt
- ¼ cup raw cacao powder
- ¼ teaspoon raw honey
- ½ teaspoon vanilla
- ¼ teaspoon ground cinnamon

Directions:
1. Add walnuts and almonds to the food processor and blend until finely ground.
2. Add dates to nut mix and continue to process for about 2 minutes.
3. Place remaining ingredients into the food processor and blend until combined and smooth.
4. Roll dough into 1 tablespoon sized balls and chill in the fridge for at least 2 hours before serving.

366 - Coconut Raspberry Bites

Servings: 2
Total Time: 10 minutes (optional 2 hours chilling)

Ingredients:
- ½ cup almond meal
- 4 dates, pitted, soaked for 15 minutes then drained
- ½ cup unsweetened, shredded coconut, divided
- ¾ cup freeze-dried raspberries, divided
- ¼ cup cacao powder
- 3 tablespoons coconut butter, melted
- 3 tablespoons maple syrup
- 1 teaspoon vanilla extract
- ½ teaspoon Himalayan salt
- ¼ cup cacao nibs

Directions:
1. Combine almond meal, dates, half of the shredded coconut, half of the raspberries, cacao powder, coconut butter, maple syrup, vanilla and salt in a food processor until smooth.
2. Add in remaining coconut, raspberries and the cacao nibs. Pulse a few times so that these are incorporated but not entirely smooth.
3. Roll dough into 1 tablespoon size balls.
4. Either serve immediately or chill for 2 hours in the fridge before serving.

367 - Double Chocolate Cookie Dough Bites

Servings: 2
Total Time: 10 minutes plus 2 hours chilling

Ingredients:
- 1 cup oats
- 1 cup raw almonds
- ½ teaspoon salt
- ¼ teaspoon cinnamon
- 1 tablespoon vanilla extract
- 3 tablespoons maple syrup
- 2 tablespoons coconut oil, melted
- ¼ cup raw cacao powder
- ½ cup chickpeas, cooked
- 2 tablespoons cacao nibs

Directions:
1. In a food processor or high speed blender, add oats, almonds, salt, cinnamon and vanilla extract. Blend until a flour-like consistency is formed.
2. Add in maple syrup, coconut oil, cacao and chickpeas. Blend until smooth and a dough forms.
3. Stir in cacao nibs. Form into 1 tablespoon sized balls and chill for 2 hours before serving.

368 - Buckwheat Chocolate Crepe Cake

Servings: 2
Total Time: 35 minutes

Ingredients:
- 2 tablespoons ground flaxseeds
- 6 tablespoons water
- 1 cup buckwheat flour
- 1 tablespoon coconut oil, melted
- ½ teaspoon Himalayan salt
- ½ teaspoon coconut sugar
- ½ teaspoon vanilla extract
- ¼ teaspoon cinnamon
- ¼ cup raw cacao powder
- 2 cups water
- 2 tablespoons ghee, melted

Whipped Coconut Cream

- 1 can full fat coconut milk, chilled overnight in the fridge
- ½ teaspoon vanilla extract
- ½ teaspoon lemon zest
- 1 tablespoon maple syrup

Directions:
1. To prepare Coconut Whipped Cream, open the can of coconut milk and drain the water for later use. Add coconut cream to a bowl (preferably a chilled metal bowl) and add the vanilla, zest and maple syrup. Beat with a hand mixer for 3 minutes or until fluffy.
2. In a small bowl, whisk together ground flaxseeds and water. Place in the freezer for 15 minutes or until a gel forms.
3. In a blender, combine flaxseeds mixture, buckwheat, coconut oil, salt, sugar, vanilla, cinnamon, cacao and 2 cups water. Blend well and set aside.
4. Brush ghee on a medium nonstick skillet and place over medium-low heat. Add some of the batter to pan and swirl around entire pan to create even layer. Cook 3 minutes on each side. Remove and repeat until batter is finished.
5. On a plate, place a crepe and top with some of the Whipped Coconut Cream. Place another crepe on top and repeat again with Whipped Coconut Cream. Continue layering until all the crepes are used.
6. Run a knife around the edge of the cake to clean any extra cream, slice into wedges and serve.

369 - Cashew Chip Cookies

Servings: Makes 4-5 large cookies
Total Time: 25 minutes

Ingredients:
- ½ can garbanzo beans, drained and rinsed
- 1 teaspoon vanilla extract
- ¼ cup cashew butter
- ¼ cup honey
- ½ teaspoon baking powder
- ⅛ teaspoon Himalayan salt
- 1/3 cup vegan chocolate chips or cacao chips

Directions:
1. Preheat oven to 350°F/175°C. Line a baking tray with parchment paper.
2. Add all ingredients except the chocolate chips (or cacao chips) to a food processor and blend until smooth.
3. Roll dough into 4-5 balls and press down on the balls with a fork on the baking tray.
4. Bake in the oven for 10-15 minutes or until slightly browned.

370 - Pineapple Ice Cream

Servings: 2
Total Time: 15 minutes plus 2 hours of freeze time minimum

Ingredients:
- 1 ½ cups pineapple, cubed
- ½ cup coconut water
- 2 dates, pitted and soaked 15 minutes then drained
- ¼ teaspoon vanilla extract
- ⅛ teaspoon Himalayan salt
- ½ cup coconut milk
- 1/3 cup coconut cream
- 1 lime, zested and juiced

Directions:
1. Place pineapple, coconut water, dates, vanilla and salt in a food processor or blender and process until well combined.
2. Transfer to a medium sized bowl and add the coconut milk, coconut cream, lime juice and lime zest. Stir well to combine.
3. Transfer to ice cream maker and process according to manufacturer's instructions. Alternatively, pour into a freezer-safe dish and freeze, stirring vigorously every 30 minutes until frozen and then freezing for 2 hours.
4. If using the ice cream maker, transfer mixture to freezer-safe dish and freeze for 2 hours.

---

371 - Mixed Fruit Tart

Servings: Makes 8 tarts
Total Time: 20 minutes plus 1 hour chilling

Ingredients:
- ½ cup raw almonds
- ¼ cup raw walnuts
- ¼ cup unsweetened shredded coconut
- ½ cup dates, pitted and quartered
- 2 tablespoons cup melted coconut oil
- ⅛ teaspoon Himalayan salt
- ⅛ teaspoon nutmeg
- ⅛ teaspoon cinnamon

Filling

- 1 ½ ounces raspberries
- 1 ½ ounces blackberries
- ¼ cup dates, pitted and quartered
- 1 tablespoon melted coconut oil
- 1 tablespoon lemon juice
- ⅛ teaspoon Himalayan salt

<u>Topping</u>

- 3 ounces raspberries
- 3 ounces blackberries
- 1 tablespoon raw honey
- 1 tablespoon mint, chopped

Directions:
1. In a food processor, combine the almonds and walnuts until a flour-like consistency starts to form. Add coconut, dates, oil, salt, nutmeg and cinnamon. Process until a dough forms.
2. Press dough into a small tart pan and chill in fridge while you make the filling.
3. Clean the food processor.
4. Combine all the Filling ingredients in the food processor and blend until smooth. Pour into the prepared crust and chill for 1 hour.
5. Top with raspberries, blackberries, and lightly drizzle honey and along with the chopped mint.

372 - Chocolate Orange Cheesecake

Servings: 2
Total Time: 20 minutes plus 1 hour and 30 minutes freezing time

Ingredients:
- ½ cup walnuts
- ½ cup almonds
- ¾ cup dates, pitted
- 1 tablespoon raw cacao
- ½ teaspoon vanilla
- ⅛ teaspoon Himalayan salt
- 1 tablespoon orange zest

Filling

- ½ cup raw cashews, soaked overnight, rinsed and drained
- 1 tablespoon maple syrup
- ¼ teaspoon vanilla
- 4 ounces full-fat coconut milk
- ½ tablespoon lemon juice
- 1 tablespoon orange juice
- 1 teaspoon orange zest
- 1 tablespoon raw cacao
- 1 tablespoon coconut oil, melted
- ¼ teaspoon Himalayan salt
- ⅛ teaspoon cinnamon

Directions:
1. In a food processor, combine the walnuts and almonds until crumbly consistency is reached. Add in dates, cacao, vanilla and salt. Process until a dough forms.
2. Press dough into two individual tart shells and place in the freezer for 15 minutes.
3. While crust is in the freezer, make the Filling by combining all the Filling ingredients in a food processor or blender until smooth.
4. Remove tart shells from the freezer and pour Filling into each. Freeze for 15 minutes and then sprinkle orange zest on top.
5. Chill in the fridge for another 1 hour before serving.

373 - Summer Crumble

Servings: 2
Total Time: 50 minutes

Ingredients:
- 1 cup peaches, sliced
- ¾ cup raspberries
- 1 teaspoon coconut oil
- 1 tablespoon coconut sugar
- 1 teaspoon ginger, grated
- 1 teaspoon lemon juice
- 1 tablespoon arrowroot starch

Crumble Topping

- 1 ½ tablespoons water
- 1/3 cup coconut sugar
- 2 tablespoons coconut oil
- ⅛ teaspoon Himalayan salt
- ⅛ teaspoon cinnamon
- ½ teaspoon vanilla extract
- ½ teaspoon almond extract
- ¼ cup walnuts, chopped
- 2 tablespoons oats
- ¼ cup unsweetened, shredded coconut

Directions:
1. Preheat oven to 375°F/190°C.
2. In a small glass baking dish, combine peaches, raspberries, oil, sugar, ginger, lemon juice and arrowroot. Toss well to coat evenly. Bake in the oven for 15 minutes.
3. While the fruit bakes, make the Crumble Topping by heating water in a medium skillet over medium heat until it comes to a low boil. Add coconut sugar and stir until dissolved. Reduce heat to low and simmer for 2 minutes before adding the oil, salt, cinnamon, vanilla extract and almond extract.
4. Remove skillet from the heat and stir in walnuts, oats and shredded coconut. Drop Crumble Topping all over the peach and blueberry mixture, making sure it is well covered.
5. Bake in the oven for another 15-20 minutes and remove.
6. Let cool 5 minutes before serving.

374 - Cauliflower Rice Pudding

Servings: 2
Total Time: 45 minutes

Ingredients:
- 2 tablespoons flaxseeds
- 6 tablespoons water
- ¼ head cauliflower, cut into florets (will make about ½ cup rice)
- 2 tablespoons raw honey
- ¼ teaspoon sea salt
- 2 tablespoons arrowroot
- ½ cup raisins
- ½ teaspoon vanilla extract
- ¼ teaspoon almond extract
- 2 cups unsweetened coconut milk
- ¼ teaspoon cinnamon
- ¼ teaspoon nutmeg
- ⅛ teaspoon ground cloves

Directions:
1. Preheat oven to 350°F/175°C.
2. In a small bowl, whisk together the flaxseeds and water. Set aside in the fridge for 10 minutes until a gel forms.
3. Place cauliflower in a food processor and pulse a few times to create the cauliflower rice.
4. Add the cauliflower rice, flaxseeds gel, honey, salt, arrowroot, raisins, vanilla, almond, coconut milk, cinnamon, nutmeg and cloves to a medium sized bowl and combine well.
5. Pour the mixture from the bowl into a small glass baking dish and bake in the oven for 30 minutes.
6. Remove from oven and serve immediately.

375 - Raw Coconut Lemon Cookies

Servings: Makes approx. 6 cookies
Total Time: 15 minutes plus 1 hour chill time

Ingredients:
- 1/3 cup cashews
- ½ cup almond meal
- 4 dates, pitted, soaked 10 minutes and drained
- 1 cup (+ 2 tablespoons) unsweetened, shredded coconut
- 1 ½ tablespoons lemon juice
- 1 tablespoon coconut butter
- 1 teaspoon lemon zest

Directions:
1. Place cashews in the food processor and pulse until a fine flour-like texture forms. Add in almond meal, dates, 1 cup coconut, lemon juice and coconut butter and process until a dough forms.
2. On a small plate combine 2 extra tablespoons of coconut with lemon zest.
3. Roll dough into tablespoon sized balls and roll each ball in the coconut and lemon mixture.
4. Place balls on a plate and let chill in the fridge for 1 hour.

376 - Lemon Lime Jelly Dessert

Servings: 2
Total Time: 15 minutes plus 1 hour chill time

Ingredients:
- ¼ teaspoon agar agar powder
- ¼ cup water
- ¼ cup coconut milk
- ⅛ teaspoon lime extract
- ⅛ teaspoon lemon extract
- 1 tablespoon honey
- ½ teaspoon lime zest
- ½ teaspoon lemon zest
- ½ cup diced kiwi

Directions:
1. In a medium-sized saucepan, dissolve agar agar in half of the water and let stand for 5 minutes.
2. While agar agar mixture stands, heat coconut milk in a small saucepan over medium-low heat. After 5 minutes, heat agar agar mixture over low heat while stirring constantly.
3. When agar agar mixture comes to a low boil, pour the warmed coconut milk, lime extract, lemon extract, honey, lime zest and lemon zest in with the agar agar mixture. Stir well and let cook for 4 minutes.
4. Remove from heat and pour into desired mold.
5. Let chill in the fridge for at least 1 hour before removing from the mold and topping with kiwi.

377 - Gingered Pear Bowl

Servings: 1
Total Time: 10 minutes

Ingredients:
- 2 pear, cored and cubed
- 2 tablespoons fresh ginger, grated
- 1 teaspoon cinnamon
- 1 teaspoon Himalayan salt
- 1 tablespoon walnuts, toasted and crushed

Yogurt Sauce

- 1 tablespoon unsweetened yogurt
- 1 teaspoon maple syrup
- ¼ teaspoon nutmeg

Tahini Sauce

- 1 tablespoon tahini
- 1 teaspoon maple syrup
- 1 teaspoon warm water
- ½ teaspoon cinnamon
- ¼ teaspoon Himalayan salt

Directions:
1. Place pear, ginger, cinnamon, salt and walnuts in a regular sized eating bowl and set aside.
2. In a small bowl, prepare the Yogurt Sauce by combining the Yogurt Sauce ingredients together.
3. In another small bowl, prepare the Tahini Sauce by combining the Tahini Sauce ingredients together.
4. Spoon the Yogurt Sauce and Tahini Sauce over the pears and serve.

---

378 - Strawberry Coconut Lime Bites

Servings: Makes 6 bites
Total Time: 10 minutes plus 30 minutes chill time

Ingredients:
- 6 tablespoons unsweetened, shredded coconut
- 2 teaspoons lime zest
- ⅛ teaspoon Himalayan salt
- ¼ cup coconut butter, melted
- 6 strawberries

Directions:
1. On a small plate, combine the shredded coconut, lime zest and salt
2. Take a small spoonful of the coconut butter and press it up against a strawberry. You may need to spread it around the strawberry with your fingers.
3. Roll the strawberry in the coconut lime mixture.
4. Repeat with the remaining strawberries.
5. Set on a large plate and chill in the fridge for at least 30 minutes before serving.

---

379 - Coconut Chip Bites

Servings: Makes 8 bites
Total Time: 25 minutes

Ingredients:
- 1 very ripe banana, mashed
- 2/3 cup unsweetened, shredded coconut
- 1 teaspoon coconut flour
- ¼ teaspoon vanilla extract
- ⅛ teaspoon Himalayan salt
- 1 teaspoon cacao nibs

Directions:
1. Preheat oven to 350°F/175°C. Line a baking tray with parchment paper.
2. Combine all the ingredients in a large bowl. Mix thoroughly until dough-like texture is created.
3. Spoon dough into 6 balls on the tray and press down on each ball.
4. Bake in the oven for 10-15 minutes or until they are lightly browned.

380 - Sweet Potato Orange Cookies

Servings: Makes 12 cookies
Total Time: 35 minutes

Ingredients:
- ¾ cup mashed sweet potato
- 1/3 cup quick oats
- 1 tablespoon cashew butter
- 1 egg
- 1 ½ tablespoon honey
- 1 teaspoon orange blossom water
- ¼ teaspoon vanilla
- ¼ teaspoon cinnamon
- ⅛ teaspoon nutmeg
- ¼ teaspoon baking powder
- ¼ teaspoon baking soda
- ⅛ teaspoon Himalayan salt
- 1 teaspoon orange zest
- 1 tablespoon raisins

Directions:
1. Preheat oven to 350°F/175°C. Line a baking tray with parchment paper.
2. Add all the ingredients, except the raisins to a food processor and blend until combined. Fold in raisins.
3. Scoop 12 balls of dough onto the baking tray. Flatten with a fork and bake for 20 minutes, flipping once halfway through.
4. Remove and let cool before serving.

381 - Cashew Coconut Cold Cookies

Servings: Makes 10 cookies
Total Time: 15 minutes plus 30 minutes chill time

Ingredients:
- 1/3 cup unsweetened, shredded coconut
- 1/3 cup gluten-free rolled oats
- 1 tablespoon ground flaxseed
- 2 tablespoons cashews, finely ground
- 1/3 cup cashew butter
- 2 tablespoons maple syrup
- 1 teaspoon cacao nibs
- ¼ teaspoon Himalayan salt

Directions:
1. In a large bowl, combine all ingredients until a dough forms.
2. Roll 10 pieces of dough into a ball and place on a plate.
3. Chill 30 minutes before serving.

382 - Pumpkin Cups

Servings: 1
Total Time: 5 minutes plus 8 hours chill time

Ingredients:
- 1 cup unsweetened almond milk
- 2 tablespoons chia seeds
- ½ teaspoon ground ginger
- ½ teaspoon ground cinnamon
- ¼ teaspoon ground nutmeg
- 1 tablespoon pure maple syrup
- ½ cup pumpkin puree
- ½ teaspoon vanilla extract
- 1 teaspoon flaxseed, ground
- 1 teaspoon unsweetened, shredded coconut
- 1 tablespoon pecans, crushed

Directions:
1. Combine all ingredients, except coconut and pecan in a large drinking glass (that has a cover) or a jar. Make sure combined thoroughly.
2. Cover and set in the fridge for at least 8 hours.
3. Garnish with coconut and pecans before serving.

383 - Strawberry Roll Ups

Servings: 2
Total Time: 5 minutes plus 4 hours cook time

Ingredients:
- 1 cup strawberries, hulled and chopped
- ½ cup unsweetened applesauce
- 3 soft pitted dates

Directions:
1. Preheat oven to 200°F/95°C. Line a baking tray with parchment paper.
2. Combine all the ingredients in a food processor or blender.
3. Pour the mixture onto the baking tray, spread it out into a thin layer and bake in the oven for 4 hours.
4. Remove and cut into strips to roll up

---

384 - Pumpkin Pie & Cacao Fudge

Servings: 2
Total Time: 25 minutes plus 2 hours chill time

Ingredients:
- ½ cup sunflower butter
- 2 tablespoons coconut oil
- ¼ cup pumpkin puree
- ½ teaspoon ground ginger
- ½ teaspoon ground cinnamon
- ¼ teaspoon ground nutmeg
- 1 tablespoon maple syrup
- 2 tablespoons cacao nibs

Directions:
1. Line a small glass baking dish with parchment paper.
2. In a small saucepan over medium-low heat, melt sunflower butter and coconut oil. Stir in pumpkin puree, ginger, cinnamon, nutmeg and maple syrup. Keep occasionally stirring for about 15-20 minutes.
3. Remove from heat and fold in cacao nibs.
4. Pour mixture into the baking dish and place in the fridge until firm, at least 2 hours.

---

385 - Strawberry & Lime Balls

Servings: 2
Total Time: 5 minutes plus 30 minutes chill time

Ingredients:
- 1/3 cup cashews
- ¾ cup shredded coconut
- ¼ cup diced strawberries
- 1 tablespoon maple syrup
- 1 lime, juiced
- 2 teaspoons lime zest
- 2 ½ tablespoons almond flour
- ½ teaspoon pure vanilla extract
- 2 tablespoons melted coconut oil

Directions:
1. Process the cashews in a food processor until a flour forms. Add the rest of the ingredients to the food processor and combine.
2. Roll dough into small balls and place on a baking tray lined with parchment paper.
3. Place in the freezer for at least 30 minutes before serving.

---

386 - Papaya Popsicles

Servings: 2
Total Time: 5 minutes plus 4 hours freeze time

Ingredients:
- ½ cup papaya, chopped
- ½ pineapple, chopped
- ¼ cup light coconut milk
- ½ cup coconut water
- 1 tablespoon raw honey
- 2 limes, zested and juiced
- 1 orange, juiced

Directions:
1. Combine all the ingredients in a blender and pour into popsicle molds.
2. Place in the freezer for at least 4 hours.

387 - Lemon Cashew Coated Strawberries

Servings: 2
Total Time: 10 minutes plus 1 hour chill time

Ingredients:
- 1 cup raw cashews, soaked in cold water for 4 hours then drained and rinsed
- 1 cup pitted dates, pitted and soaked in cold water for 4 hours, drained and rinsed
- 1 tablespoon vanilla extract
- ¼ teaspoon almond extract
- 1 teaspoon lemon juice
- 1 teaspoon lemon zest
- ¼ teaspoon cinnamon
- 1 tablespoon unsweetened almond milk
- 1 pint of fresh strawberries, washed, dried, tops sliced off and middle scooped out
- 2 tablespoons mint, finely chopped

Directions:
1. In a food processor, combine the cashews, dates, vanilla, almond extract, lemon juice, lemon zest, cinnamon and almond milk until smooth.
2. Spoon cashew mixture into each of the strawberries.
3. Sprinkle mint on the top of the strawberry.
4. Chill for 1 hour before serving.

388 - Chai Tahini Ice Cream

Servings: 2
Total Time: 5 minutes plus 4 hours freeze time

Ingredients:
- 1 can full fat coconut milk
- 1 tablespoon maple syrup
- ½ cup tahini
- ½ teaspoon ground cardamom
- ¼ teaspoon ground cinnamon
- ¼ teaspoon ground ginger
- ¼ teaspoon ground cloves

Directions:
1. Place all the ingredients in a blender and mix until smooth.
2. Pour mixture into small, freezer-safe bowl and freeze at least 4 hours.

389 - Apricot Crumble

Servings: 2
Total Time: 40 minutes

Ingredients:
- 1 tablespoon coconut oil
- 5 apricots, coarsely chopped
- ½ cup raspberries
- 1 tablespoon chia seeds
- 1 tablespoon ginger, grated
- 1 tablespoon honey
- 1 cup rolled oats
- ½ cup ground almonds
- ¼ cup sliced almonds
- 1 tablespoon sunflower seeds
- ¼ cup unsweetened, shredded coconut
- ¼ cup maple syrup
- ¼ cup melted coconut oil
- ½ teaspoon salt
- ¼ teaspoon cinnamon

Directions:
1. Preheat oven to 350°F/175°C. Grease a small glass baking dish with 1 tablespoon of coconut oil.
2. In a large bowl, combine the apricots and raspberries with the chia seeds, ginger and honey. Pour into the baking dish and set aside.
3. Add the oats, ground almonds, sliced almonds, sunflower seeds, coconut, maple syrup, ¼ cup coconut oil, salt and cinnamon to the large bowl. Combine well so that entire mixture is moistened with the oil and syrup.
4. Sprinkle oats mixture over the apricot and raspberry mixture.
5. Bake in the oven for 30 minutes.
6. Remove and let cool 5 minutes before serving.

390 - Chocolate Sea Salt Popsicles

Servings: 2
Total Time: 5 minutes plus 4 hours freeze time

Ingredients:
- 1 large ripe avocado
- ½ cup full fat coconut milk
- 2 tablespoons maple syrup
- ¼ cup raw cacao powder
- ¼ teaspoon flakey sea salt
- ⅛ teaspoon cinnamon

Directions:
1. Combine all ingredients in a blender until smooth.
2. Pour mixture into popsicle mold and freeze in the freezer for at least 4 hours.

---

391 - Summer Fruit Mold

Servings: 2
Total Time: 15 minutes plus 3 hours rest time

Ingredients:
- ¼ cantaloupe, seeds removed and cut into small balls with melon baller
- ¼ honeydew melon, seeds removed and cut into small balls with melon baller
- ¼ cup raspberries
- 1 cup fresh apple juice
- ¼ cup water
- 2 tablespoons agar agar flakes
- 2 tablespoons honey

Directions:
1. Place cantaloupe balls, melon balls and the raspberries in a mini loaf pan.
2. Bring apple juice, water and agar agar to a boil in a medium saucepan over medium-low heat. Make sure the agar agar is dissolved, this will take about 5 minutes.
3. Remove from heat and stir in the honey. Cover the saucepan and let cool.
4. Pour mixture over the melon and raspberries in the mini loaf pan.
5. Let set 3 hours on the counter.
6. Place on a plate and flip over when ready to serve.

---

392 - Baked Pears with Whipped Coconut Cream

Servings: 2
Total Time: 50 minutes

Ingredients:
- 1 forelle pear, halved and cored
- 1 cinnamon stick, halved lengthwise
- ½ vanilla bean, halved lengthwise and widthwise
- 1 teaspoon ginger, grated
- 2 tablespoons golden raisins
- 2 tablespoons currants
- 1 lemon, zested
- 1 teaspoon coconut oil
- ¼ cup water

Whipped Coconut Cream (Optional)

- 1 can full fat coconut milk, chilled overnight in the fridge
- ½ teaspoon vanilla extract
- ¼ teaspoon cinnamon
- 1 tablespoon maple syrup

Directions:
1. Preheat oven to 350°F/175°C. Cut two medium-sized pieces of parchment paper and fold in half. Cut out a heart shape from the folded parchment paper.
2. Set parchment paper out in front of you and place a pear near the fold on each piece. On top of each add cinnamon stick, vanilla bean, ginger, raisins, currants, lemon zest and coconut oil. Pour a few drops of water over each.
3. Fold the edges to make overlapping folds until entire package is sealed entirely.
4. Place both on a baking tray and bake for 40 minutes.
5. To make the Whipped Coconut Cream, if using, open the can of coconut milk and drain the water for later use. Add coconut cream to a bowl (preferably a chilled metal bowl) and add the vanilla, cinnamon and maple syrup. Beat with a hand mixer for 3 minutes or until fluffy.
6. Serve pear topped with the Whipped Coconut Cream.

393 - Mango Mint Mousse Cups

Servings: 2
Total Time: 10 minutes

Ingredients:
- 2 ripe mangos
- ½ cup pineapple, cubed
- ½ banana, sliced
- 1 cup full fat coconut milk
- 1 lime, juiced and zested
- 1 teaspoon ginger, grated
- 2 tablespoons mint
- ¼ cup raspberries

Directions:
1. Combine all the ingredients, instead of the raspberries, in a blender and mix until smooth and creamy.
2. Top with raspberries and serve.

394 - Ginger Peach & Raspberry Popsicles

Servings: 2
Total Time: 5 minutes plus 4 hours freeze time

Ingredients:
- 4 peaches, peeled, pitted and chopped
- 2 teaspoons lemon juice
- 1-inch piece ginger, grated
- ½ very ripe banana
- ½ cup raspberries, diced

Directions:
1. Combine all the ingredients in a blender and combine until smooth.
2. Pour into popsicle molds and freeze for at least 4 hours.

395 - Oatmeal Banana Raisin Cookies

Servings: 2
Total Time: 30 minutes

Ingredients:
- 1 ripe bananas, mashed
- ½ cup rolled oats
- ¼ cup raisins
- ¼ teaspoon cinnamon
- ¼ teaspoon nutmeg
- ⅛ teaspoon ground cloves
- ⅛ teaspoon Himalayan salt

Directions:
1. Preheat oven to 350°F/175°C. Line a baking tray with parchment paper.
2. Combine all the ingredients in a medium bowl until well combined.
3. Drop tablespoon balls of the mixture onto prepared baking tray.
4. Bake 15 minutes or until lightly browned.
5. Let cool 10 minutes before serving.

396 - Raw Mint Chip Cookies

Servings: 2
Total Time: 10 minutes plus 30 minutes chill time

Ingredients:
- ½ cup oats
- ½ cup almonds
- ¼ cup mint
- 2 tablespoons cacao
- ½ cup dates, pitted and soaked 10 minutes then drained and rinsed
- 1 teaspoon peppermint extract
- ¼ teaspoon vanilla extract
- ¼ teaspoon Himalayan salt
- 1 teaspoon cacao nibs

Directions:
1. Place oats and almonds in food processor and combine until a fine flour forms. Add in mint and cacao and process until combined.
2. Add in dates, peppermint extract, vanilla extract and salt.
3. Process until a ball of dough forms.
4. Roll dough into tablespoon sized balls. Place balls on a plate and press down with a fork. Press a few cacao nibs into the top of each cookie.
5. Place in the fridge for at least 30 minutes before serving.

397 - Frozen Chocolate Orange Banana Pops

Servings: 2
Total Time: 10 minutes plus 1 hour freeze time

Ingredients:
- ¼ cup coconut oil, melted
- 2 tablespoons raw cacao powder
- 1 tablespoon maple syrup
- ½ teaspoon orange extract
- 2 bananas
- 1 tablespoon orange zest
- 1 tablespoon unsweetened, shredded coconut

Directions:
1. Line a baking tray with parchment paper. In a small bowl with high sides, whisk together the coconut oil, cacao, maple syrup and orange extract.
2. Place a popsicle stick into each of the bananas. Dip each banana into the chocolate mixture, rolling it around to make sure it is completely covered.
3. Place bananas on the baking tray and top with the orange zest and coconut.
4. Freeze in the freezer for at least 1 hour.

398 - Glazed Cinnamon Buns

Servings: 2
Total Time: 15 minutes plus 1 hour freeze time

Ingredients:
- 1 ½ cups almonds
- ½ cup walnuts
- 1 ½ cups dates, pitted
- 1 teaspoon vanilla
- ¼ teaspoon Himalayan salt
- 3 tablespoons cinnamon
- 1 teaspoon nutmeg
- ¼ cup almonds, slivered and divided
- 1 tablespoon raw honey
- 1 tablespoon coconut cream
- ½ tablespoon coconut butter, melted

Directions:
1. In a food processor, pulse the almonds and walnuts together until a fine flour forms. Add in dates, vanilla and salt and continue to process until incorporated.
2. Remove half of the mixture and set aside.
3. Add cinnamon and nutmeg to the food processor and process until combined. Remove remaining dough from food processor.
4. Roll out each half of the dough into equal sized rectangle. Top regular dough with ¼ of slivered almonds. Place the cinnamon nutmeg dough on top of the almond layer and press down lightly. Top with remaining slivered almonds.
5. Roll up the dough, forming a long log. Wrap in parchment paper and place in freezer for 1 hour.
6. While cinnamon roll chills, make glaze by combining the honey, coconut cream and coconut butter in a small bowl.
7. Remove cinnamon roll and slice into even slices. Drizzle glaze on top before serving.

399 - Lemon Sorbet

Servings: 2
Total Time: 10 minutes plus 5 hours freeze time

Ingredients:
- ½ cup coconut cream
- ½ cup dates, pitted, soaked overnight, drained and rinsed
- 2 tablespoons water
- 2 lemons, zested and juiced
- 1 teaspoon lemon extract
- 2 tablespoons raw honey
- ¼ cup unsweetened coconut milk
- 2 mint leaves

Directions:
1. In a high speed blender, combine all the ingredients except the mint leaves.
2. Place in a small glass baking dish and freeze 2 hours.
3. Stir mixture and freeze again for 3 more hours.
4. Scoop lemon sorbet into 2 bowls to serve.

---

400 - Raspberry Mint Cheesecake Ice Cream

Servings: 2
Total Time: 10 minutes plus 5 hours freeze time

Ingredients:
- 1 ½ cup raspberries
- ⅛ cup raw cashews, soaked overnight and drained
- 1 teaspoon lemon juice
- 1 teaspoon lemon zest
- 1 cup coconut milk
- 1 tablespoon coconut cream
- 1 teaspoon vanilla extract
- 2 dates, pitted
- ¼ cup mint, chopped

Directions:
1. Combine all ingredients in a food processor until smooth.
2. Place in a small glass baking dish and freeze 2 hours.
3. Stir and return to freezer for another 3 hours.
4. Remove and let sit 5 minutes before serving.

Conclusion

I hope you enjoyed all the delicious, but simple alkaline recipes in this cookbook!

For more simple and delicious cookbooks, be sure to check out my author page on Amazon at "Gloria Lee," as I'm constantly creating more cookbooks to accommodate those who wish to eat towards a healthier lifestyle.

If you enjoyed this cookbook and found it well worth the money for 400 recipes! Then please take the time to leave this cookbook a review on Amazon. I appreciate your honest feedback, and it really helps me to continue producing high-quality cookbooks that contain stacks of yummy recipes!

Simply visit my book listing page on Amazon to leave a review. You can do this by typing "Alkaline Diet Cookbook: 400 Recipes For Rapid Weight Loss & Balancing Your pH Levels" on Amazon or typing this URL into your browser: **www.amazon.com/dp/B07H6XKHRJ**

Otherwise, no worries! Keep eating well and living healthy!

I wish you all the best on your Alkaline Diet journey!

Printed in Great
Britain
by Amazon